iActuate:

100 day guide to complete fitness

Sheg Aranmolate, MD

INSPIVIA

Inspivia Books
Nashville, TN, 37203
www.inspivia.com

The information presented in this book is educational, and it is not in any way, shape or form meant to be a substitute for the valuable advice of your healthcare professional. It is advisable that you consult with your physician about matters concerning your health or require medical attention, and before embarking on any form of exercise, diet or medical treatment.

iActuate: 100 day guide to complete fitness

Editors – Daniel Smyth, Daniel Dorset
Cover Designer – Steve Danielson
Author Photograph – Sheg Aranmolate

ISBN-10: 0984845917
ISBN-13: 978-0-9848459-1-0

This Inspivia Books softcover edition May 2016

Inspivia Books is a trademark of Inspivia, Inc.

Manufactured in the United States of America

table of contents:

dedication:

To my darling wife for being my best friend and greatest supporter through thick and thin.

To my little ones for giving me courage and inspiring me to always pursue my dreams.

To my parents for instilling in me great morals and values.

To my sisters for being the best cheerleading team in my life.

I am Thankful.

acknowledgment:

First and foremost, I thank God for giving me the strength and knowledge to write this book.

I thank my family and friends for their encouragements, support and efforts in helping me make this book a reality.

I thank my friend, Steve Danielson, for all the time and effort he put into designing the book cover.

I thank my friend, Daniel Dorset, for meticulously proofreading the book.

Finally, I thank my friend and editor, Daniel Smyth, for all his helpful comments and criticisms.

I am Grateful.

introduction:

I finished this book at the tender age of twenty-three but recently added minor edits to reflect my maturity. While I was writing it, I was often asked for the title or the overarching idea. Like many writers, I started the project without a title in mind and had to confess as such. Nevertheless, I often told inquirers that I was writing to *actuate* people to improve their lives. Over time, I noticed that I often emphasized the words 'i" and 'Actuate," when talking about the project and so I concluded that iActuate would be a great book title. This wasn't entirely due to the convenience of the title, but rather because the title embodies my philosophy behind the book. The lowercase 'i" represents my humble self and the word 'Actuate" represents my intense desire to incite, motivate, and inspire myself and others to succeed in life. Over the course of my young life, I have learned a lot about life, justice, ethics, and morality from my brilliant parents and from the works of some of the world's great thinkers, such as Aristotle, Kant, Nietzsche, Marx, Einstein, and Soyinka. However, I believe that my life experiences have been my greatest instructor of all. Drawing from all that I've learned thus far, I wrote this collection of micro-essays to inspire people, regardless of their age, creed, or gender and to show them that we still live in a world filled with kindness and inspiration. I hope that the time readers spend with this book will be a journey for them to better understand their strengths and weaknesses and to realize that they are living sources of inspiration. I hope that by reading all the daily messages, performing the effective workouts and following the simple nutritional advice in the book, you will become healthier and more physically, mentally, and emotionally fit.

notes from the author:

Employing elements of applied psychology and physiology, I wrote this book to be simple, practical and to the point. As a result, I avoided the use of heavy scientific, theoretical and philosophical concepts that are not useful or practical to the everyday person. This book does not present you with any novel breakthroughs in the field of medicine, psychology or kinesiology as the marketplace is already filled with thousands of books and articles on such subjects. Instead, I want the contents of this book to be like the encouraging words of a good friend, personal trainer or life coach who speaks to you from experience and offers advice for your guidance and development. The book is structured like a daily fitness journal that provides you (male or female) with effective strength building workouts and exercises that target and develop the major muscle groups of the body and burn fat. The book also offers you inspirational micro-essays that provide you with logical reasons to be inspired. The simple, yet effective nutritional advice in the book is derived from the *Paleo* diet, which is based on the types of foods that early humans had eaten, consisting mostly of lean meats, fish, seafood, nuts, eggs, vegetables and fruits, and excluding dairy, sugars, grain products and processed foods. I understand that we live in a busy world and you may be tempted to read the book in its entirety at once. Although this is acceptable, I still urge you to complete the daily exercises and follow the nutritional advice in the book to achieve optimal detoxification and total transformation in one-hundred (100) days. In conclusion, this book is like a daily shot of physical and inspirational espresso to get your day to its best start!

let's get started:

☐ take a full body photo on day 1
☐ record your weight and calculate your BMI (body mass index)

day one (1):	weight (lbs):		BMI:	

BMI categories:
underweight = <18.5 | normal weight = 18.5–24.9 | overweight = 25–29.9 | obesity = ≥30

day one:
human potential

> The best and safest thing is to keep a balance in your life,
> acknowledge the great powers around us and in us. If you
> can do that, and live that way, you are really a wise man.
>
> Euripides

A while back, a young woman decided to write me for advice. She wrote me a sincere letter describing how depressed, confused and frustrated she was with her life and her family. She said her life was stagnant and it seemed like everyone except her was succeeding. She added, however, that she knew she had the potential to make a difference and change her life but just didn't know where to start. I found her letter touching and it inspired me to help her understand the concept of the 'human potential." The 'human potential" is like a corn kernel that if planted in the soil is capable of growth. However, if left unattended in the ground, then various elements like disease, pests, weeds and lack of essential nutrients will have a better chance of diminishing its growth. Every human being has a unique potential to grow and thrive, but just like the corn kernel we need continual attention, nurturing and care. It is important for us to remove those harmful habits and thoughts that constantly stunt our growth and to surround ourselves with positive ideas and positive people, similar to pulling weeds and giving a supportive environment for corn seeds to grow. Nevertheless, just as adding excessive fertilizers can be harmful to plants, excessive pressure on ourselves to develop can make us feel worthless and thus tarnish our growth. Similarly to the handling of delicate crops by a learned farmer, always treat yourself with care, detoxify yourself of bad vibes, don't be too critical of yourself, and at the end of the season you will reap the great bounty of your potential.

tasks:

☺ select a weight that provides the most resistance for every 10 reps
please keep rest interval between each rep to less than 60 seconds

workout: chest

☐ incline bench press   [10 reps x 5 times]

weights (lbs):					

☐ decline bench press   [10 reps x 5 times]

weights (lbs):					

☐ flat bench press   [10 reps x 5 times]

weights (lbs):					

☐ pec deck   [10 reps x 5 times]

weights (lbs):					

☐ hammer press   [10 reps x 5 times]

weights (lbs):					

☐ dips   [20 reps x 5 times]

weights (lbs):					

cardio: treadmill

☐ paced walk / jog   [30 minutes]

calories:	

nutrition:

☐ drink at least eight 8-ounce cups of water
☐ take a multivitamin
☐ eat only lean meats, fish, seafood, nuts, fruits and vegetables
☐ drink 1 serving of a protein shake before breakfast and dinner
☐ avoid starches, grains, sugars, juice, sweets and soda
☐ avoid all artificially colored and processed foods

day two:
in denial

No legacy is so rich as honesty.
William Shakespeare

Suppose you get into your car in the morning on your way to work, and as you are driving you notice that the fuel indicator is blinking, signifying that your car is low on gas. It is very likely that you will be on the lookout for the nearest gas station. Wouldn't it be absurd, if you saw the light blinking and happened to see a gas station ahead, but instead of stopping for gas, you concluded that the light was meaningless because you could smell gasoline in your fuel tank? Obviously, anyone who drives a car knows that this way of thinking is unwarranted and will likely result in the car stalling a few miles down the road. Denial! There are so many of us who are in denial and are always making excuses to avoid the reality of our problems. Just like the delusional driver who refuses to accept the reality that the car is out of gas, many of us are aware of our problems but continually refuse to accept that fact. We keep making up intelligent and sometimes illogical reasons why the problems we have aren't real or important. Nevertheless, we must remember that we are the true judges and the best solvers of our problems--we know them better than anyone else. Therefore, when we make those ridiculous excuses, we're not deceiving anyone but ourselves. You can't keep on making excuses for your negative actions and keep on ignoring those warning signs, because after a few miles down the path of life you will be stalled and unable to progress any further like a car without gasoline.

workout: back/traps

☐ deadlift   [10 reps x 5 times]

weights (lbs):					

☐ pulldowns   [10 reps x 5 times]

weights (lbs):					

☐ bent over row   [10 reps x 5 times]

weights (lbs):					

☐ cable row   [10 reps x 5 times]

weights (lbs):					

☐ pull ups   [10 reps x 5 times]

weights (lbs):					

☐ shrugs   [10 reps x 5 times]

weights (lbs):					

cardio: stairmaster

☐ paced walk   [30 minutes]

calories:	

nutrition:

☐ drink at least eight 8-ounce cups of water
☐ take a multivitamin
☐ eat only lean meats, fish, seafood, nuts, fruits and vegetables
☐ drink 1 serving of a protein shake before breakfast and dinner
☐ avoid starches, grains, sugars, juice, sweets and soda
☐ avoid all artificially colored and processed foods

Sheg Aranmolate, MD

day three:
our burden

Judge thyself with the judgment of sincerity, and thou will
judge others with the judgment of charity.
John Mitchell Mason

L ife is filled with its ups and downs, and many of us from a young age have been taught by society to only reveal our successes and triumphs, and to keep secret our failures and problems. As a result, many people today are walking around with many problems that they haven't shared with anyone. I understand that many of us feel that in revealing our problems to others, we might be inconveniencing them or they might lose respect for us as individuals. In fact, the reverse is usually true as good people gain respect for us when we share our problems with them. They sincerely empathize and genuinely want to help us lessen our burden. Hiding our problems is similar to a young boy receiving a bad grade on a report card, and instead of showing it to his parents who could educate him or get him proper help and tutoring, decides to hide it under his pillow. The boy assumes that his parents only want to see good grades and unwisely thinks that because the report card is out of sight, everything is all right. As expected, his teacher already recorded the bad grade and it will come back to haunt him later in the school year. Don't be like this naïve little boy who failed to reveal his problems to people who could help. If you are having problems in your life, talk to a family member or a friend, and if none of them can help, at least seek out a trained professional. Are you going to reveal your problems or are you still going to keep hiding your problems, only to be haunted by them later in life? Do what's right and let someone else help you with your burden.

---

tasks:

workout: legs

☐ squats   [10 reps x 5 times]

weights (lbs):				

☐ squat to bench   [10 reps x 5 times]

weights (lbs):				

☐ quad extensions   [15 reps x 5 times]

weights (lbs):				

☐ leg curls   [15 reps x 5 times]

weights (lbs):				

☐ leg press calf raises   [20 reps x 5 times]

weights (lbs):				

☐ seated calf raises   [20 reps x 5 times]

weights (lbs):				

cardio: elliptical

☐ paced walk   [30 minutes]

calories:	

nutrition:

☐ drink at least eight 8-ounce cups of water
☐ take a multivitamin
☐ eat only lean meats, fish, seafood, nuts, fruits and vegetables
☐ drink 1 serving of a protein shake before breakfast and dinner
☐ avoid starches, grains, sugars, juice, sweets and soda
☐ avoid all artificially colored and processed foods

Sheg Aranmolate, MD

day four:
mental compartmentalization

> When we are planning for posterity, we ought to remember
> that virtue is not hereditary.
> <u>Thomas Paine</u>

H ave you ever tried watching two movies on television at the same time--clicking back and forth between both movies? If so, you probably know that it is difficult to fully understand both movies as you are likely to miss important parts of the plots in the process. You could have avoided wasting your time and ruining your chances of enjoying both movies if you had watched one movie at a time. Interestingly, this scenario is similar to the way many of us deal with and solve problems in our lives. Instead of 'mentally compartmentalizing" our problems, and individually focusing on and solving our problems, we try to multitask and fix all our problems at once--often with little or no success. Libraries often arrange books on shelves numerically and alphabetically for easy accessibility. On the other hand, if libraries randomly placed books on selves without a filing system, finding a particular book would be much more difficult. Likewise, when it comes to sorting and solving our problems, many of us are like large unorganized libraries with randomly-scattered books. Consequently, we end up becoming inefficient and disorganized problem solvers. Efficient problem-solving requires us to continually sort our problems so that we are better able to prioritize them and tackle one problem at a time. For this reason, do your best to resolve all your office issues at work and all your household issues at home. Don't try solving both problems at the same time and place.

tasks:

workout: deltoids

☐ military press behind the neck   [10 reps x 5 times]

weights (lbs):					

☐ military press   [10 reps x 5 times]

weights (lbs):					

☐ dumbbell shoulder press   [10 reps x 5 times]

weights (lbs):					

☐ machine shoulder press   [10 reps x 5 times]

weights (lbs):					

☐ reverse pec deck   [10 reps x 5 times]

weights (lbs):					

☐ dumbbell front raises   [20 reps x 5 times]

weights (lbs):					

cardio: treadmill

☐ paced walk/jog   [30 minutes]

calories:	

nutrition:

☐ drink at least eight 8-ounce cups of water
☐ take a multivitamin
☐ eat only lean meats, fish, seafood, nuts, fruits and vegetables
☐ drink 1 serving of a protein shake before breakfast and dinner
☐ avoid starches, grains, sugars, juice, sweets and soda
☐ avoid all artificially colored and processed foods

Sheg Aranmolate, MD

day five:
fear of change

> Great ability develops and reveals itself increasingly with
> every new assignment.
> Baltasar Gracian

I remember the first time a friend invited me on a snowboarding trip: because I grew up in a country devoid of snow, I wanted to ensure that it was a memorable trip. I began making plans months ahead. I read up on snowboarding and Salt Lake City, Utah, bought several pieces of snowboarding gear, and by the time of the trip I felt prepared to have fun. However, even with all this anticipation, when I got to the mountaintop and saw the large vastness of all the snow below, my excitement turned to fear. I became so scared that I didn't want to snowboard at all. In all honesty, do you think that my fears were valid or do you think that I was just a scared loser unable to proceed? The truth is that many of us, at some point, want to do new things like visit exotic places, live in new cities or change jobs. But we can easily become apprehensive when given the opportunity to do these things. The initial fear of change is normal because these activities require us to leave our comfort zone and venture into unknown territories. You need to realize that feeling scared of change doesn't make you a coward. In fact, it can make you a more vigilant and heedful person. On the other hand, if you simply succumb to your fears, then you might miss out on great life experiences. When I was on the mountaintop and was about to give up snowboarding, I thought about how much time and energy I had invested in preparing for the trip that I realized that quitting wasn't an option. In such times of apprehension and doubt, remember that you aren't a coward for feeling that way. Nevertheless, you shouldn't let your fears take advantage of you. Go out today and do those things that you have always wanted to do.

workout: arms/forearms

☐ pushdowns   [10 reps x 5 times]

weights (lbs):					

☐ wide grip curls   [10 reps x 5 times]

weights (lbs):					

☐ single arm cable kickbacks   [10 reps x 5 times]

weights (lbs):					

☐ seated triceps press   [10 reps x 5 times]

weights (lbs):					

☐ hammer curls   [10 reps x 5 times]

weights (lbs):					

☐ concentration curls   [20 reps x 5 times]

weights (lbs):					

cardio: stairmaster

☐ paced walk   [30 minutes]

calories:	

nutrition:

☐ drink at least eight 8-ounce cups of water
☐ take a multivitamin
☐ eat only lean meats, fish, seafood, nuts, fruits and vegetables
☐ drink 1 serving of a protein shake before breakfast and dinner
☐ avoid starches, grains, sugars, juice, sweets and soda
☐ avoid all artificially colored and processed foods

Sheg Aranmolate, MD

day six:
the answers within

I can't understand why people are frightened of new ideas.
I'm frightened of the old ones.
John Cage

A Greek king gave Archimedes, a great mathematician, the task of determining the quality of a gold crown that the king had recently acquired. This task was difficult for Archimedes because he didn't have any of today's sophisticated tools and techniques to determine the purity of gold. He thought long and hard about all the possible ways to solve his problem, but couldn't devise a viable solution. Resigned to report his failure to the king, Archimedes decided to take a bath before heading to the palace. As he submerged himself in the bathwater, he suddenly realized that the buoyancy of water could be used to measure the purity of gold! The point of this story is that so many of us feel that we have problems too difficult to be fixed and tasks too daunting to be resolved. As a result, we often lose hope. Ironically, as in the case of Archimedes, the solutions to our alleged problems are usually relatively simple. Unlike Archimedes, however, we never discover these solutions because we're not immersed in the right environment, or perhaps because we're too distracted to listen to the answers from within ourselves. Next time you are about to give up on an idea, task, ambition or aspiration because you don't have a solution, take some time off, go to a quiet place, and listen to your inner voice. You might be surprised to find that the solution to your problems is directly in front of you.

workout: abs/core

☐ weighted sit ups   [20 reps x 5 times]

weights (lbs):					

☐ weighted cable crunch   [10 reps x 5 times]

weights (lbs):					

☐ leg raises   [20 reps x 5 times]

weights (lbs):					

☐ air bike   [60 reps x 5 times]

weights (lbs):					

☐ side bends   [40 reps x 5 times]

weights (lbs):					

☐ hanging leg raises   [20 reps x 5 times]

weights (lbs):					

cardio: elliptical

☐ paced walk   [30 minutes]

calories:	

nutrition:

☐ drink at least eight 8-ounce cups of water
☐ take a multivitamin
☐ eat only lean meats, fish, seafood, nuts, fruits and vegetables
☐ drink 1 serving of a protein shake before breakfast and dinner
☐ avoid starches, grains, sugars, juice, sweets and soda
☐ avoid all artificially colored and processed foods

day seven:
panic attack

> Let the fear of danger be a spur to prevent it; he that fears
> not, gives advantage to the danger.
>
> <u>Francis Quarles</u>

The 'victim with the keys" is a classic scene that I often see repeated in several scary and horror movies. This scene usually depicts a scared individual running away from a killer or a monster towards a room or a car that represents their freedom or salvation. Adding to the suspense, these individuals get to the door, pull out a bunch of keys, and begin to fumble them in search for the right key. Unfortunately, these already terrified people then begin to panic, wasting time, as they frantically try to open the door, only to be captured or hurt by their assailants. This classic movie scene can be similar to moments in our lives, especially when we are confronted with physical, financial, or emotional difficulties. During these times, it usually seems like every time we get close to our door of salvation, things always go wrong and we end up getting beaten by our problems. Of note, many of us seem to forget that we have in our possession, in the form of great ideas, the keys to set ourselves free--called solutions. However, like those people in the classic movie scene, we become so overwhelmed that we fail to find the correct key (solution) from the bunch. Whenever you feel like you are being pursued by life's problems, and when you sense that you are close to your door of salvation, don't panic because anxiety only makes things worse. Instead, try to relax, take control, find the correct key (solution), and open the door to your financial, emotional, physical and spiritual freedom.

workout: none
- ☐ rest

cardio: none
- ☐ rest

nutrition:
- ☐ drink at least eight 8-ounce cups of water
- ☐ take a multivitamin
- ☐ eat only lean meats, fish, seafood, nuts, fruits and vegetables
- ☐ drink 1 serving of a protein shake before breakfast and dinner
- ☐ enjoy sugars, juice, sweets and soda in moderation
- ☐ avoid all artificially colored and processed foods

Sheg Aranmolate, MD

day eight:
ideal happiness

> Happiness depends upon ourselves.
> Aristotle

During my course in life as a personal fitness trainer, I had the opportunity to work with people from various walks of life and to learn the truth that money doesn't always equate to happiness. For example, I remember a wealthy client of mine who owned a business, drove a luxury car, owned a nice home in an expensive neighborhood, and had no problem spending money. However, after working with him and getting to know him, I realized that he was depressed and even suicidal. According to himself, despite all the money at his disposal, he had no reason to love life. There are many people in the world who are in a similar position as my client. These people are financially successful, and seem to be happy and content with life. Other people see them and wish they had their wonderful lives. The unfortunate truth is that a number of these people are pretenders who in public seem to have it all, but behind closed doors are living wretched unhappy lives. Be careful of what you wish for in life because you might get it, only for you to realize that it's nothing like what you wanted. Don't wish to be happy like someone else, because we truly never know the entire truth about a person. Instead, gradually develop yourself into a person that embodies and pursues happiness in the right places, such as by helping others, spending time with family and friends, exercising and learning. Be careful not to think riches will give you happiness or can solve all your problems. If you're not already a happy person, no amount of money in this world can change that fact about you.

tasks:

workout: chest

☐ incline bench press   [10 reps x 5 times]

weights (lbs):					

☐ decline bench press   [10 reps x 5 times]

weights (lbs):					

☐ flat bench press   [10 reps x 5 times]

weights (lbs):					

☐ pec deck   [10 reps x 5 times]

weights (lbs):					

☐ hammer press   [10 reps x 5 times]

weights (lbs):					

☐ dips   [20 reps x 5 times]

weights (lbs):					

cardio: treadmill

☐ paced walk/jog   [30 minutes]

calories:	

nutrition:

☐ drink at least eight 8-ounce cups of water
☐ take a multivitamin
☐ eat only lean meats, fish, seafood, nuts, fruits and vegetables
☐ drink 1 serving of a protein shake before breakfast and dinner
☐ avoid starches, grains, sugars, juice, sweets and soda
☐ avoid all artificially colored and processed foods

day nine:
a little kindness

> Forget injuries, never forget kindnesses.
> Confucius

A few years ago, I was in Lagos, Nigeria and there was a period of widespread poverty, high unemployment, and food scarcity mainly because corrupt politicians poorly governed the country and siphoned most of the country's wealth for personal use. It was a truly difficult and devastating period for several families, and I vividly remember that many people were starving, unable to afford healthy meals and basic human necessities. Sadly and quite sorry to say, a large number of merchants and wealthy individuals who had access to stored food supplies began to increase the prices of food items to ensure that they made astronomical gains at the expense of the poor and impoverished. On the other hand, a few generous and kindhearted individuals offered discounts on food supplies to families and sometimes gave out free food to the famished. It is undeniable that businesses thrives on the idea of making a profit for every sale, but during times when human lives are at stake making huge profit margins should be the least important issue. In times of despair, when many people are dependent on each other for survival will you be a selfish opportunist like those merchants who jacked up their prices? Or will you be a selfless philanthropist, striving to share joy and happiness to the less fortunate? Kindness and altruistic behaviors may not always be financially profitable, but in the grand scheme of life these gestures are invaluable to humanity. Become a philanthropist today in your own way and change someone's life for the better.

workout: back/traps

☐ deadlift   [10 reps x 5 times]

weights (lbs):					

☐ pulldowns   [10 reps x 5 times]

weights (lbs):					

☐ bent over row   [10 reps x 5 times]

weights (lbs):					

☐ cable row   [10 reps x 5 times]

weights (lbs):					

☐ pull ups   [10 reps x 5 times]

weights (lbs):					

☐ shrugs   [10 reps x 5 times]

weights (lbs):					

cardio: stairmaster

☐ paced walk   [30 minutes]

calories:	

nutrition:

☐ drink at least eight 8-ounce cups of water
☐ take a multivitamin
☐ eat only lean meats, fish, seafood, nuts, fruits and vegetables
☐ drink 1 serving of a protein shake before breakfast and dinner
☐ avoid starches, grains, sugars, juice, sweets and soda
☐ avoid all artificially colored and processed foods

day ten:
fading away

> To win without risk is to triumph without glory.
> Pierre Corneille

One day I was in a café drinking a cup of tea and happened to strike up a conversation with an attractive young woman. We started talking about politics but suddenly started talking about her life. She told me that she used to be a successful fashion model but had recently decided to go back to college to become a teacher. She said she mainly did this out of fear of fading away into oblivion without making a positive difference in the world. Upon hearing her story, I immediately could relate with this woman because every one of us as we mature through life will at some point have the fear or feeling of fading away through time without genuine accomplishments. The different stages in our lives are similar to the chapters of a book, with each chapter marking a new beginning but a continuation of previous chapters. Just as every chapter in an action novel isn't filled with action sequences, every stage in our lives won't be marked by continuous recognition. There are times when we will be popular and there are times when we will not. There are times when we win and there are times when we fail. Also, there are times when we just need to relax and build up experience to do those things that really matter to us. It is important to realize that as long as we are breathing, there should be no reason for anyone to be scared of fading away. This fear is only a state of mind--to reverse its effects we need to prove to ourselves that we are not fading away. Go out today and find something that makes you feel good about yourself. Remember the world is filled with endless possibilities and the limit of your sky is dependent on how high you are willing to fly.

workout: legs

☐ squats   [10 reps x 5 times]

weights (lbs):				

☐ squat to bench   [10 reps x 5 times]

weights (lbs):				

☐ quad extensions   [15 reps x 5 times]

weights (lbs):				

☐ leg curls   [15 reps x 5 times]

weights (lbs):				

☐ leg press calf raises   [20 reps x 5 times]

weights (lbs):				

☐ seated calf raises   [20 reps x 5 times]

weights (lbs):				

cardio: treadmill

☐ paced walk/jog   [30 minutes]

calories:	

nutrition:

☐ drink at least eight 8-ounce cups of water
☐ take a multivitamin
☐ eat only lean meats, fish, seafood, nuts, fruits and vegetables
☐ drink 1 serving of a protein shake before breakfast and dinner
☐ avoid starches, grains, sugars, juice, sweets and soda
☐ avoid all artificially colored and processed foods

day eleven:
the right attention

> Love is the difficult realization that something other than
> oneself is real.
> Iris Murdoch

At some point, you might have noticed that parents with toddlers usually have a tough time shopping in a store. It seems like every time these parents begin to look at store items their toddlers get fussy and upset because their parents aren't giving them undivided attention. Babies and toddlers, despite their sometimes extreme demands for affection, reveal two basic human features: our desire for attention and signs of approval from other people, and our disappointment when we don't get that needed attention. I once heard the story of a brilliant professor at a prestigious university who had worked diligently for several years. One day, he was found dead in his office. His apparent suicide note revealed that he killed himself because nobody cared about how he felt, only about how much he could contribute to the university. This story is sad because that institution lost a bright individual at least in part because it failed to show appreciation to its faculty. It is easy for us to get caught up in the webs of our society and fail to show our appreciation to people around us. All the same, you might be surprised to find that a few kind words of appreciation and encouragement can do a lot of good. Take some time out of your busy life and compliment someone else. You never know--your kind words might be the difference between life and death.

tasks:

workout: deltoids

☐ military press behind the neck   [10 reps x 5 times]

weights (lbs):					

☐ military press   [10 reps x 5 times]

weights (lbs):					

☐ dumbbell shoulder press   [10 reps x 5 times]

weights (lbs):					

☐ machine shoulder press   [10 reps x 5 times]

weights (lbs):					

☐ reverse pec deck   [10 reps x 5 times]

weights (lbs):					

☐ dumbbell front raises   [20 reps x 5 times]

weights (lbs):					

cardio: treadmill

☐ paced walk/jog   [30 minutes]

calories:	

nutrition:

☐ drink at least eight 8-ounce cups of water
☐ take a multivitamin
☐ eat only lean meats, fish, seafood, nuts, fruits and vegetables
☐ drink 1 serving of a protein shake before breakfast and dinner
☐ avoid starches, grains, sugars, juice, sweets and soda
☐ avoid all artificially colored and processed foods

day twelve:
exemplar

> Reputation is what other people know about you. Honor is
> what you know about yourself.
> <u>Lois McMaster Bujold</u>

You know what? A young and upcoming physicist is most likely mentored by a venerated physics professor. A young basketball player probably looks up to an older player for inspiration. A young actor usually mimics older well-established actors--the list keeps on going. The truth is that regardless of what path we decide to pursue in life, we tend to have role models that we look up to for advice and inspiration. In an intriguing way, many of us become like our role models over time and tend to incorporate many of their fundamental values into our lives. Therefore, it is important for us to always look up to positive role models, not negative ones. On several occasions, I have had several people ask me for my source of inspiration and the power that drives me to succeed in life. I tell them that although my passion for success comes from within, I get my inspiration from positive role models. Furthermore, I tell them that whenever I decide to try something new in life, I find people who have excelled in doing it and strive to become as successful. Sometimes, I even imagine that these people are always judging my actions. All this makes me act appropriately and work harder. Who do you look up to? Is it your parents, your teacher, your professor, a celebrity or an athlete? Whoever it is, will this person be impressed by your work ethic and the way you treat others, or will they be disappointed? Think about the way your role models will react to your actions. Also remember that someone else might be looking up to you for inspiration, so always act appropriately towards others and be positive.

tasks:

workout: arms/forearms

☐ pushdowns   [10 reps x 5 times]

weights (lbs):					

☐ wide grip curls   [10 reps x 5 times]

weights (lbs):					

☐ single arm cable kickbacks   [10 reps x 5 times]

weights (lbs):					

☐ seated triceps press   [10 reps x 5 times]

weights (lbs):					

☐ hammer curls   [10 reps x 5 times]

weights (lbs):					

☐ concentration curls   [20 reps x 5 times]

weights (lbs):					

cardio: stairmaster

☐ paced walk   [30 minutes]

calories:	

nutrition:

☐ drink at least eight 8-ounce cups of water
☐ take a multivitamin
☐ eat only lean meats, fish, seafood, nuts, fruits and vegetables
☐ drink 1 serving of a protein shake before breakfast and dinner
☐ avoid starches, grains, sugars, juice, sweets and soda
☐ avoid all artificially colored and processed foods

Sheg Aranmolate, MD

day thirteen:
talkative ones

Toil to make yourself remarkable by some talent or other.
Seneca

Nowadays, there is an unspoken rule about having a cell phone, and it seems taboo not to have one. It's becoming really bad these days because many of us are becoming very condescending towards people who don't own cell phones. More and more of us are becoming so attached to our phones that a day without it feels like being lost in the wilderness. It is also uncommon these days for a person to have a phone plan without unlimited nights and weekend minutes, and funny enough, many us actually do take advantage of these plans. In fact, if unlimited talk could be quantified, many of us will have talked innumerable times over the phone to converse about trivial issues. Please don't get me wrong as it is good to call and talk to our family and friends, and to check on their wellbeing. However, when we start gossiping about others and spreading hateful thoughts and messages, then our phone talk becomes useless. It is quite unfortunate that many of us have already spent what amounts to several days of our lives on the phone or internet with nothing tangible to show for them, days we could have spent making a difference in our lives and in other people's lives. Have you ever taken the time to listen to your typical phone conversation? You might be surprised to find out that some of your conversations are empty and you could have better used the time you spent on those conversations for more constructive activities. It is more likely that careless talk will bring you more trouble than peace. Thus, be careful of what you say, how you say it, and when you say it. Don't be like those annoying individuals on the bus or in the store, who talk loudly on their cell phones about nothing important, letting their valuable talents go to waste.

tasks:

workout: abs/core

☐ weighted sit ups   [20 reps x 5 times]

weights (lbs):					

☐ weighted cable crunch   [10 reps x 5 times]

weights (lbs):					

☐ leg raises   [20 reps x 5 times]

weights (lbs):					

☐ air bike   [60 reps x 5 times]

weights (lbs):					

☐ side bends   [40 reps x 5 times]

weights (lbs):					

☐ hanging leg raises   [20 reps x 5 times]

weights (lbs):					

cardio: elliptical

☐ paced walk   [30 minutes]

calories:	

nutrition:

☐ drink at least eight 8-ounce cups of water
☐ take a multivitamin
☐ eat only lean meats, fish, seafood, nuts, fruits and vegetables
☐ drink 1 serving of a protein shake before breakfast and dinner
☐ avoid starches, grains, sugars, juice, sweets and soda
☐ avoid all artificially colored and processed foods

day fourteen:
gratefulness

> Gratitude is born in hearts that take time to count up past
> mercies.
> Charles E. Jefferson

O nce, I happened to be watching a television show about investors buying and selling homes for profit. It was exciting to see people 'flipping" homes at fast rates and making sizable profits. These investors buy old homes, fix them up in a few weeks, and sell them for a profit. Yet, I noticed that many of these investors got upset whenever they sold a home lower than their initial asking price. The feeling of disappointment in these individuals is normal because they didn't get what they wanted. On the contrary, they failed to realize that things could have been much worse for them. For instance, they could have lost the home to a fire or a natural disaster, just to mention a few calamities. The drive to become highly successful is great to have, but many of us sometimes get carried away with this desire that we become ungrateful and forgetful of all the good things around us. When we don't get the results that we want, it is important to always be thankful for our many blessings and to realize that life could be worse. Funny enough, many of us don't realize that the ability to complain about life is a luxury in itself. There are millions of people around the world who live in miserable conditions and don't have the luxury to complain about it. Take some time out of your busy life and drive to the nearby children's hospital. You will be saddened to see how much pain and suffering some little children endure everyday without complaining. Simply be thankful for the breath of life.

tasks:

workout: none
☐ rest

cardio: none
☐ rest

nutrition:
☐ drink at least eight 8-ounce cups of water
☐ take a multivitamin
☐ eat only lean meats, fish, seafood, nuts, fruits and vegetables
☐ drink 1 serving of a protein shake before breakfast and dinner
☐ enjoy sugars, juice, sweets and soda in moderation
☐ avoid all artificially colored and processed foods

Sheg Aranmolate, MD

day fifteen:
cool it

An unhurried sense of time is in itself a form of wealth.
<u>Bonnie Friedman</u>

What time is it? This is a typical question that you probably have been asked by someone else, and it is one of the few questions to which you and the several billion other people in the world can relate. We always want to know the time because we have all of our activities invested in time. We pay our bills based on certain times of the month, we get paid according to how much time we spend working, and we celebrate special occasions based on certain times of the year. I was recently watching a movie and I heard an interesting statement about time, which suggested that time is simply a series of numbers with attached meanings, and without these meanings time is nothing more than numbers. In all actuality, this description of time is correct. Time is a concept that was developed by humans, using numbers to keep track of events, and we indeed give these otherwise meaningless numbers power. Many of us have become so engulfed by time that we literally have become slaves to it. Our every move and action is determined by the time, and many of us can't function without knowing the time. We have become like addicts in that we allow our fast paced and time-conscious lifestyles to ruin our personal relationships. Of course, it will be ridiculous for anyone to completely ignore the time; however, it is important for us take some time off each day to breathe and recuperate. Use this period to think about and appreciate all those wonderful things around us, like our family, friends, pets, good food, scenic landscapes, and escape to a place where we can relax and forget about all the worries we have attached to time.

---

workout: chest

☐ incline bench press   [10 reps x 5 times]

weights (lbs):					

☐ decline bench press   [10 reps x 5 times]

weights (lbs):					

☐ flat bench press   [10 reps x 5 times]

weights (lbs):					

☐ pec deck   [10 reps x 5 times]

weights (lbs):					

☐ hammer press   [10 reps x 5 times]

weights (lbs):					

☐ dips   [20 reps x 5 times]

weights (lbs):					

cardio: treadmill

☐ paced walk/jog   [30 minutes]

calories:	

nutrition:

☐ drink at least eight 8-ounce cups of water
☐ take a multivitamin
☐ eat only lean meats, fish, seafood, nuts, fruits and vegetables
☐ drink 1 serving of a protein shake before breakfast and dinner
☐ avoid starches, grains, sugars, juice, sweets and soda
☐ avoid all artificially colored and processed foods

day sixteen:
rage

When anger rises, think of the consequences.
Confucius

I was watching the television one morning and happened to catch a news exclusive that focused on the aftermath of a tornado storm on a small town. The tornado had literally destroyed the entire town and its important landmarks. The schools, libraries, shops and all other important buildings were all in pieces, and I remember watching several of the town members cry and lament on how quickly the tornado had destroyed their homes. These people's lamentations, in a unique way, got me thinking about anger and its damaging effects. The repercussion of our anger can very much be like a wild tornado, rapidly advancing through a town and producing tremendous, irreversible damage along the way. There are so many us who have seriously hurt ourselves and our loved ones because we let our anger take control of our actions. Our anger burst usually begins with someone or something ticking us off and then suddenly we unleash our severely damaging 'inner tornado." Do you remember the last time you got angry? Did you say or do things that you normally will not say or do? Did you hurt people that you wouldn't normally hurt? Anger is a powerful emotion that can destroy and has destroyed many great people. Remember that just as nature controls the occurrence of tornadoes, we have the ability to control our actions, even when we're angry. Hence, next time someone angers you, take a moment to think about all the damage that could result if you let your anger get the best of you.

tasks:

workout: back/traps

☐ deadlift   [10 reps x 5 times]

weights (lbs):					

☐ pulldowns   [10 reps x 5 times]

weights (lbs):					

☐ bent over row   [10 reps x 5 times]

weights (lbs):					

☐ cable row   [10 reps x 5 times]

weights (lbs):					

☐ pull ups   [10 reps x 5 times]

weights (lbs):					

☐ shrugs   [10 reps x 5 times]

weights (lbs):					

cardio: stairmaster

☐ paced walk   [30 minutes]

calories:	

nutrition:

☐ drink at least eight 8-ounce cups of water
☐ take a multivitamin
☐ eat only lean meats, fish, seafood, nuts, fruits and vegetables
☐ drink 1 serving of a protein shake before breakfast and dinner
☐ avoid starches, grains, sugars, juice, sweets and soda
☐ avoid all artificially colored and processed foods

Sheg Aranmolate, MD

day seventeen:
my deadline

> Nothing is stronger than habit.
> <u>Ovid</u>

Deadlines! Everyday of our lives, we are confronted with one deadline or another. Nowadays, it seems like every aspect of our lives has a deadline, from our tasks at work, to our bills at home, to our assignments at school. We all know from experience that failure to meet these deadlines usually results in some type of penalty. The fear of being penalized is for the most part the driving force that motivates many of us to complete our tasks. In fact, so many of us have become so accustomed to deadlines that we can't function optimally without some sort of deadline. Let's assume that your boss at work gave you two days to complete an important task that affected the entire structure of your company. It is quite obvious that if you wanted to keep your job, you will work really hard to complete the task in the allotted time. It's ironic that many of us strive to complete deadlines set by others but fail to complete deadlines set by ourselves. I have worked with a number of people who frequently set personal deadlines for themselves, such as living a healthy lifestyle, joining a gym or even ditching a bad habit. However, these individuals never accomplished their goals or aspirations. The reason many of us fail to meet our personal deadlines is because we don't get penalized upon failure. To get around this problem, we need to hold ourselves accountable for our actions and penalize ourselves whenever we fail to meet our deadlines. You will be amazed how this mentality will motivate and help you accomplish your set goals. Quit failing and letting yourself down! Take better care of your life and remember that your personal deadlines are at least as important as any other deadline.

tasks:

workout: legs

☐ squats   [10 reps x 5 times]

weights (lbs):				

☐ squat to bench   [10 reps x 5 times]

weights (lbs):				

☐ quad extensions   [15 reps x 5 times]

weights (lbs):				

☐ leg curls   [15 reps x 5 times]

weights (lbs):				

☐ leg press calf raises   [20 reps x 5 times]

weights (lbs):				

☐ seated calf raises   [20 reps x 5 times]

weights (lbs):				

cardio: elliptical

☐ paced walk   [30 minutes]

calories:	

nutrition:

☐ drink at least eight 8-ounce cups of water
☐ take a multivitamin
☐ eat only lean meats, fish, seafood, nuts, fruits and vegetables
☐ drink 1 serving of a protein shake before breakfast and dinner
☐ avoid starches, grains, sugars, juice, sweets and soda
☐ avoid all artificially colored and processed foods

day eighteen:
more junk

> Junk is the ultimate merchandise. The junk merchant does
> not sell his product to the consumer, he sells the consumer
> to the product. He does not improve and simplify his
> merchandise, he degrades and simplifies the client.
> William S. Burroughs

Whenever I walk into a thrift store, I always get amazed by the large amounts of 'stuff" that are up for sale and by the fluctuation between the ratio of items that I consider to be valuable and those that I consider to be worthless. These observations clearly confirm that there is a constant interchange between donated and purchased items. It also strengthens the adage that one person's trash is another person's treasure. It is without question that humans have a constant thirst for 'stuff," especially material stuff, and we are always out to replace or replenish our old 'stuff" with more 'stuff," either old or new. Along the same lines, there's no doubt that we live in a material world and it is unfortunate that many of us have become so engulfed by all the materialism that we tend to forget the important aspects of life that really matter, such as our family, our friends and good relationships with people. Have you ever had the chance to visit an estate auction? If so, then you know that all the material things we acquire during our lifetime will do us no good at the time of our demise. I don't, in any way, imply that we should suffer and experience life without material pleasures. However, we should be more in-tune with ourselves and more conscious of the people around us so that we don't miss out on the truly beautiful aspects of life. Remember that true friendship is more important and valuable than any riches in the world. Riches vanish with time, but true friendship strengthens with each passing day.

tasks:

workout: deltoids

☐ military press behind the neck   [10 reps x 5 times]

weights (lbs):					

☐ military press   [10 reps x 5 times]

weights (lbs):					

☐ dumbbell shoulder press   [10 reps x 5 times]

weights (lbs):					

☐ machine shoulder press   [10 reps x 5 times]

weights (lbs):					

☐ reverse pec deck   [10 reps x 5 times]

weights (lbs):					

☐ dumbbell front raises   [20 reps x 5 times]

weights (lbs):					

cardio: treadmill

☐ paced walk/jog   [30 minutes]

calories:	

nutrition:

☐ drink at least eight 8-ounce cups of water
☐ take a multivitamin
☐ eat only lean meats, fish, seafood, nuts, fruits and vegetables
☐ drink 1 serving of a protein shake before breakfast and dinner
☐ avoid starches, grains, sugars, juice, sweets and soda
☐ avoid all artificially colored and processed foods

day nineteen:
always be primed

> In preparing for battle I have always found that plans are
> useless, but planning is indispensable.
> <u>Dwight D. Eisenhower</u>

Sometimes, when I am done shopping in the mall and happen to have some idle time, I head towards the food court to eat and relax my aching feet. During those times, I watch the actions and behaviors of several people in the mall. There are the window-shoppers who gaze randomly in awe, the causal shoppers who are easily distracted by sale items, and the resolute shoppers who always seem to be rushed and determined. I have noticed that each of these different types of shoppers, despite occupying the same space, all seem to be driven by the same thing: impulsivity. Though some are more blatant than others, the fact remains that the choices and actions of these people are motivated by the lights, the sale signs and several other compelling features within the mall. No doubt we can be sporadic and spontaneous in our choices and actions. This characteristic can be good, such as when it comes to artistic creativity. However, it can also be a deterrent, like when we need to make important life decisions. Once I talked to a young woman who had recently graduated from college. Unlike most graduates who are elated about graduation, she was frustrated because she felt she had chosen her major on impulse and graduated with a degree that she disliked. Many of us are like this woman because we become sad and depressed after making impulsive choices that become grave mistakes. 'Buyer's remorse" is the common term for it. It is important to realize, however, that regardless of any impulsive choice you have made, what's done is done and you can't let your mistakes hold you captive. Learn from those mistakes, move on with your life, and always be prepared for your next big decision. All this will help you to avoid making impulsive decisions.

---

workout: arms/forearms

☐ pushdowns   [10 reps x 5 times]

weights (lbs):					

☐ wide grip curls   [10 reps x 5 times]

weights (lbs):					

☐ single arm cable kickbacks   [10 reps x 5 times]

weights (lbs):					

☐ seated triceps press   [10 reps x 5 times]

weights (lbs):					

☐ hammer curls   [10 reps x 5 times]

weights (lbs):					

☐ concentration curls   [20 reps x 5 times]

weights (lbs):					

cardio: stairmaster

☐ paced walk   [30 minutes]

calories:	

nutrition:

☐ drink at least eight 8-ounce cups of water
☐ take a multivitamin
☐ eat only lean meats, fish, seafood, nuts, fruits and vegetables
☐ drink 1 serving of a protein shake before breakfast and dinner
☐ avoid starches, grains, sugars, juice, sweets and soda
☐ avoid all artificially colored and processed foods

day twenty:
our legacy

> With regard to excellence, it is not enough to know, but we
> must try to have and use it.
> Aristotle

When a person retires, they are usually honored with some sort of acknowledgment ceremony and the retiree becomes replaced by a successor. However, the story of a once-brilliant professor whose retirement didn't fit the norm got me thinking about the importance of our legacy. It appears that this professor was once a respected scholar whose scientific and intellectual contributions were invaluable. However, as years passed he began to abuse alcohol, which severely interfered with his social and intellectual abilities. Despite his alcohol abuse, he wasn't fired because of his brilliance and the terms of his academic tenure. Nevertheless, a couple more years of boozing led the university to force him into an 'early retirement." On a sad note, as soon as he retired the university closed his office and never filled his position because he had already been replaced long before he left. It is an unfortunate fact that intelligent individuals sometimes make grave mistakes and embark on the path towards self-destruction. It's also a pity that because we live in a somewhat hostile world, people remember some of us (like this professor) for our failures, not all our great successes. Therefore, it is important that we avoid placing ourselves in compromising positions that tarnish our reputation and focus on our given tasks so that when we do vacate our jobs, our presence will be missed and a replacement will be desperately needed. Please don't be the reason why everyone around you is stagnant. Always give your best so that at the end of your stay you have a legacy for your successors to follow. Furthermore, show compassion to those people who are in pain and in their sadness seek outlets that often end in tragedy. If you are a troubled individual, please seek immediate help.

workout: abs/core

☐ weighted sit ups   [20 reps x 5 times]

weights (lbs):					

☐ weighted cable crunch   [10 reps x 5 times]

weights (lbs):					

☐ leg raises   [20 reps x 5 times]

weights (lbs):					

☐ air bike   [60 reps x 5 times]

weights (lbs):					

☐ side bends   [40 reps x 5 times]

weights (lbs):					

☐ hanging leg raises   [20 reps x 5 times]

weights (lbs):					

cardio: elliptical

☐ paced walk   [30 minutes]

calories:	

nutrition:

☐ drink at least eight 8-ounce cups of water
☐ take a multivitamin
☐ eat only lean meats, fish, seafood, nuts, fruits and vegetables
☐ drink 1 serving of a protein shake before breakfast and dinner
☐ avoid starches, grains, sugars, juice, sweets and soda
☐ avoid all artificially colored and processed foods

day twenty - one:
the philanthropist

> The excellence of a gift lies in its appropriateness rather than in its value.
> Charles Dudley Warner

Once, a man was at a meeting and before it started, the attendees were asked to introduce themselves. One by one, each person began by stating his or her name, age and profession. When it was this man's turn to speak, he introduced himself and said that he was a philanthropist by profession. As expected, at this announcement, he heard people in the room chuckle, and one guy in the group said, 'come on, you're not a philanthropist, what do you really do for a living?" The guy's question was sincere yet unfortunate because, like several other people in attendance, he still had a narrow conception of a philanthropist, probably a wealthy, older individual who for altruistic reasons donates money to carefully chosen charities or sets up a foundation. Ironically, there are plenty of wealthy individuals who donate to charity on a regular basis, solely for opportunistic reasons. In brief, a true philanthropist is anyone who constantly strives to benefit and better humanity, and you don't have to be a millionaire or billionaire to be one; you simply need to possess a genuine desire to help others. On an interesting note, the concept of philanthropy is relative to the recipient. For instance, a starving homeless man will consider you a bigger philanthropist than a well-to-do person would if you gave him a hot, delicious meal. The truth is that philanthropy doesn't have anything to do with how much money you have in the bank, rather how much affection you have in your heart. Don't be one of those people who reinforce the philanthropist stereotype. Instead, be a good example and show others that you don't have to be extremely rich to make a difference in another person's life. Become a philanthropist today and make your world, no matter how small or large, a better place for others to inhabit.

tasks:

workout: none
☐ rest

cardio: none
☐ rest

nutrition:
☐ drink at least eight 8-ounce cups of water
☐ take a multivitamin
☐ eat only lean meats, fish, seafood, nuts, fruits and vegetables
☐ drink 1 serving of a protein shake before breakfast and dinner
☐ enjoy sugars, juice, sweets and soda in moderation
☐ avoid all artificially colored and processed foods

Sheg Aranmolate, MD

day twenty - two:
walking away

> Strong reasons make strong actions.
> William Shakespeare

Sometimes, many of us don't realize or seem to forget that a lot of our actions, both good and bad, are directly influenced by our external environment. For example, if you walked into a restaurant and the host at the door immediately gave you a nasty attitude, it is likely that you will immediately be ticked-off and you will respond rudely as well before departing. Likewise, if the host's initial response was polite and friendly, even if you were already upset or having a crappy day you will likely respond politely as well. The truth is that we often allow other people to define our actions and determine the way we feel. Funny enough, we pride ourselves on our possession and ability to exercise free will, but we often don't utilize this innate ability and let other people dictate the way we feel. Take a moment to think about the last time you became upset or angry. Was it solely your own doing or was it the result of someone else imposing their actions and emotions on you? In all honesty, there are very few reasons why we should place ourselves in a position that allows others to determine the way we feel or act. We can be a lot more peaceful with ourselves and with the people around us if we consciously take control of our emotions and avoid mimicking other people's negative actions. Thus, next time someone talks or acts rudely towards you, instead of getting all fired up, respond politely and walk away. At the end of the day, you will be astonished by the peaceful outcomes from exercising your free will.

workout: chest

☐ incline bench press   [10 reps x 5 times]

weights (lbs):					

☐ decline bench press   [10 reps x 5 times]

weights (lbs):					

☐ flat bench press   [10 reps x 5 times]

weights (lbs):					

☐ pec deck   [10 reps x 5 times]

weights (lbs):					

☐ hammer press   [10 reps x 5 times]

weights (lbs):					

☐ dips   [20 reps x 5 times]

weights (lbs):					

cardio: treadmill

☐ paced walk/jog   [30 minutes]

calories:	

nutrition:

☐ drink at least eight 8-ounce cups of water
☐ take a multivitamin
☐ eat only lean meats, fish, seafood, nuts, fruits and vegetables
☐ drink 1 serving of a protein shake before breakfast and dinner
☐ avoid starches, grains, sugars, juice, sweets and soda
☐ avoid all artificially colored and processed foods

day twenty - three:
paranoid

> Guilt is anger directed at ourselves--at what we did or did
> not do.
> Peter McWilliams

Remember when you were a child and your parents told you not touch or play with a particular household item because it was fragile or expensive. Nevertheless, as soon as your parents weren't around, you disobeyed and played with it, only to end up breaking it like they had predicted. Then shortly afterwards you become scared of being caught and frantically tried to hide the damage. Every time your parents were nearby, your heart began to pound out of fear of being 'busted." This sudden behavioral change is simply the effects of our guilt taking a psychological toll on us. It is quite astonishing that this situation occurs in adults as well. Unlike children, who are usually guilty of issues that involve disobedience, adults are usually guilty of issues that involve trust. The typical adult guilt trip begins when we say or do hurtful things to others behind their backs. Because of our guilt, we become angry, defensive and even paranoid. We tend to automatically assume that everyone will act similarly to ourselves and we feel that everyone knows our dirty secrets. Relax! It's impossible for everyone to know all those hurtful things we might have done to others and not everyone is going to act like we did. Guilt is a powerful emotion that can make the sanest of people insane. The next time you are feeling guilty for your actions, don't let it consume you: instead tell the truth to the person you hurt. You actually might be surprised that the consequences of telling the truth are far less severe than the torment from your guilt. Don't become consumed by the paranoia of your guilt, just let it all out!

workout: back/traps

☐ deadlift   [10 reps x 5 times]

weights (lbs):					

☐ pulldowns   [10 reps x 5 times]

weights (lbs):					

☐ bent over row   [10 reps x 5 times]

weights (lbs):					

☐ cable row   [10 reps x 5 times]

weights (lbs):					

☐ pull ups   [10 reps x 5 times]

weights (lbs):					

☐ shrugs   [10 reps x 5 times]

weights (lbs):					

cardio: stairmaster

☐ paced walk   [30 minutes]

calories:	

nutrition:

☐ drink at least eight 8-ounce cups of water
☐ take a multivitamin
☐ eat only lean meats, fish, seafood, nuts, fruits and vegetables
☐ drink 1 serving of a protein shake before breakfast and dinner
☐ avoid starches, grains, sugars, juice, sweets and soda
☐ avoid all artificially colored and processed foods

day twenty - four:
different seasons

In these matters the only certainty is that nothing is certain.
Pliny the Elder

I t should come as no surprise to anyone that the weather varies with the seasons. Where I live, summer is characterized by high daily temperatures and bright sunshine. Autumn has high winds and falling leaves. Winter is usually filled with snow and low temperatures, while spring brings beautiful flowers and an abundance of bright green shoots. We realize that no matter where we live, seasonal changes are natural occurrences and consequently we don't get bothered by these changes. In fact, many of us will become worried and anxious if this normal cycle was in any way interrupted. Our lives are seasonal like the weather. As a result, there are times when life is relatively easy and times when it becomes tough. However, because many of us usually fail to realize the impermanent nature of our problems, we usually become elated during good times and saddened when the going gets rough. Every season in nature can be comfortable or uncomfortable depending on how well one is dressed. For example, if you wore warm clothes during the summer and light clothes during the winter, you will be uncomfortable in both situations because you're wearing inappropriate clothing. Similarly, in life we need to dress ourselves with the correct 'emotional clothes" to tackle the different seasons in our lives. Are you going through tough times in your life? Do they seem never-ending? These moments, like the weather, are temporary and will soon be over. Always ensure that you have the right mindset and correct gear when you tackle the rough seasons of life while, of course, enjoying the good seasons.

---

workout: legs

☐ squats   [10 reps x 5 times]

weights (lbs):				

☐ squat to bench   [10 reps x 5 times]

weights (lbs):				

☐ quad extensions   [15 reps x 5 times]

weights (lbs):				

☐ leg curls   [15 reps x 5 times]

weights (lbs):				

☐ leg press calf raises   [20 reps x 5 times]

weights (lbs):				

☐ seated calf raises   [20 reps x 5 times]

weights (lbs):				

cardio: elliptical

☐ paced walk   [30 minutes]

calories:	

nutrition:

☐ drink at least eight 8-ounce cups of water
☐ take a multivitamin
☐ eat only lean meats, fish, seafood, nuts, fruits and vegetables
☐ drink 1 serving of a protein shake before breakfast and dinner
☐ avoid starches, grains, sugars, juice, sweets and soda
☐ avoid all artificially colored and processed foods

day twenty - five:
grumbler

> Perfection is a road, not a destination. Every time I live, I get an
> education.
> Burk Hudson

I t is normal for us to sometimes feel unaccomplished, especially when we compare our lives to highly successful people in the world who have achieved so much. Without trivializing our own accomplishments, we must realize that these feelings can trigger us to pursue greater success. However, constantly worrying about the measure of our achievements can eventually become a serious problem. I have been fortunate to have the opportunity to speak with several successful people and I have noticed that these people always have a positive outlook on life, never worry excessively, and have an inextinguishable drive to succeed through good and bad times. I often get disheartened when I hear people complain that their inability to succeed in life is primarily due to such things as their gender, race, or background. The undeniable truth is that every one of us has the ability to become successful in some sense, but many of us often become stalled in life because of excuses. Take ants, for example. Compared to humans, ants are small, weak and dumb. Nevertheless, these insects never quit doing their duties like gathering food or building their ant colony. Each ant, in doing so, becomes successful in helping fellow ants. In the future, whenever you are feeling worthless or intimidated by a daunting task, take a moment to think about busy ants in the woods and how much they accomplish daily. As mentioned above, we are much bigger and smarter than ants, so we really have few legitimate excuses for not pursuing success. We must strive to banish the thoughts of complacency and start working towards our desired ambitions.

---

tasks:

workout: deltoids

☐ military press behind the neck   [10 reps x 5 times]

weights (lbs):					

☐ military press   [10 reps x 5 times]

weights (lbs):					

☐ dumbbell shoulder press   [10 reps x 5 times]

weights (lbs):					

☐ machine shoulder press   [10 reps x 5 times]

weights (lbs):					

☐ reverse pec deck   [10 reps x 5 times]

weights (lbs):					

☐ dumbbell front raises   [20 reps x 5 times]

weights (lbs):					

cardio: treadmill

☐ paced walk/jog   [30 minutes]

calories:	

nutrition:

☐ drink at least eight 8-ounce cups of water
☐ take a multivitamin
☐ eat only lean meats, fish, seafood, nuts, fruits and vegetables
☐ drink 1 serving of a protein shake before breakfast and dinner
☐ avoid starches, grains, sugars, juice, sweets and soda
☐ avoid all artificially colored and processed foods

day twenty - six:
over the limit

> Never exceed your rights, and they will soon become
> unlimited.
> <u>Jean Jacques Rousseau</u>

Whenever we walk into an elevator, the first thing we usually do is look at the left or right-hand side for the elevator buttons. However, there are several other features in the elevator that many of us don't always seem to notice such as the fire warning signs and the elevator weight limit. The law requires every elevator to place a legible sign that shows the weight limit and the maximum number of people that can be carried at a particular instance. You don't need to have an advanced physics degree to realize that it will be dangerous to operate any elevator once the maximum weight limit is exceeded because the consequences can be disastrous. In a strange and intriguing way, our temperament is like an elevator with set weight limits. If you have entered several elevators, it is quite obvious that different elevators have different weight capacities, and as a result some elevators can carry more people than others. On a similar note, some of us are able to handle larger emotional loads than others. Nonetheless, we all have our limits, and just like in the elevators these limits are often ignored or unnoticed by others. Perhaps due to our nonchalant attitude, we tend to push others--especially our loved ones--until they snap and collapse like an unstable bridge or a faulty elevator car. Please be compassionate and pay more attention to other people's emotional threshold. You don't want to continue to push others over their emotional limits, just like you will not want others to test your capacity.

workout: arms/forearms

☐ pushdowns   [10 reps x 5 times]

weights (lbs):					

☐ wide grip curls   [10 reps x 5 times]

weights (lbs):					

☐ single arm cable kickbacks   [10 reps x 5 times]

weights (lbs):					

☐ seated triceps press   [10 reps x 5 times]

weights (lbs):					

☐ hammer curls   [10 reps x 5 times]

weights (lbs):					

☐ concentration curls   [20 reps x 5 times]

weights (lbs):					

cardio: stairmaster

☐ paced walk   [30 minutes]

calories:	

nutrition:

☐ drink at least eight 8-ounce cups of water
☐ take a multivitamin
☐ eat only lean meats, fish, seafood, nuts, fruits and vegetables
☐ drink 1 serving of a protein shake before breakfast and dinner
☐ avoid starches, grains, sugars, juice, sweets and soda
☐ avoid all artificially colored and processed foods

day twenty - seven:
speak out

> The people who are the most bigoted are the people who
> have no convictions at all.
> G. K. Chesterton (1874 - 1936)

Suppose you were taking a walk around your neighborhood and suddenly, as you passed a tree, you heard the sound of a child in distress. Immediately, you look behind the trees and to your surprise or dismay you find an older child torturing an adorable toddler. Any adult in their right mind will be stunned by the older child's actions and would immediately stop the child from inflicting anymore pain on the toddler. Some might even go further, taking the toddler away from the older child and reporting the incident to the parents of both children if they happen to know them. This response to such a situation is due to our sense of justice, which is aroused by the sight of injustice and gives us an incentive to correct such unfairness. On many occasions, however, many of us fail to utilize this authority when it comes to situations that directly affect our comfort and happiness. Why do many of us continuously allow others to take advantage of our weaknesses and mistreat us on a daily basis without ever voicing our opinions? There are times in our lives when we will be mistreated like the toddler, but unfortunately there may not be anyone but ourselves to defend us. Therefore, it is important for us to learn how to stand up against such tyranny and abuse. Today, not tomorrow, is your day of liberation from those bad habits as well as demeaning and oppressive individuals who consciously or subconsciously try to humiliate you. Peacefully stand up against the oppression and let your voice be heard!

tasks:

workout: abs/core

☐ weighted sit ups   [20 reps x 5 times]

weights (lbs):				

☐ weighted cable crunch   [10 reps x 5 times]

weights (lbs):				

☐ leg raises   [20 reps x 5 times]

weights (lbs):				

☐ air bike   [60 reps x 5 times]

weights (lbs):				

☐ side bends   [40 reps x 5 times]

weights (lbs):				

☐ hanging leg raises   [20 reps x 5 times]

weights (lbs):				

cardio: elliptical

☐ paced walk   [30 minutes]

calories:

nutrition:

☐ drink at least eight 8-ounce cups of water
☐ take a multivitamin
☐ eat only lean meats, fish, seafood, nuts, fruits and vegetables
☐ drink 1 serving of a protein shake before breakfast and dinner
☐ avoid starches, grains, sugars, juice, sweets and soda
☐ avoid all artificially colored and processed foods

Sheg Aranmolate, MD

day twenty - eight:
intricate connections

> The greatest friend of Truth is time, her greatest enemy is
> Prejudice, and her constant companion Humility.
> <u>Charles Caleb Colton</u>

I f you have ever watched a documentary that depicts wild beasts like lions, tigers and antelopes in their natural habitat, then you realize that these animals on a daily basis are constantly battling the harsh elements in nature. These documentaries tend to reveal the complex interactions between different animals, especially when it comes to feeding. This network of complex interactions in biology is called the 'food web," where all animals on earth are directly or indirectly connected to each other by their desire to feed. In accordance, the large and ferocious meat-eating lion is in the end dependent on grass for continued existence because lions eat many animals that in turn depend on grass for survival. As a result, without grass, the herbivorous animals that lions eat will all die from starvation and without these animals lions will also be on their way to extinction. Humans, similarly, coexist in a world with intricate connections, whereby the input of many people from different walks of life is required for the proper functioning of our society. It is sad that many of us get carried away by our status and forget how we are all dependent on each other. For example, the auto-mechanic needs the doctor on sick days, the doctor needs the mechanic to fix his or her car, and the doctor needs the janitor to have clean hospitals and safely perform his job. Even more so, think about those nasty drivers who cut you off in traffic. You might not immediately realize it, but you are indeed dependent on those persons to pay their taxes! You shouldn't be obnoxious about your status, and instead make a conscious decision today to start treating everyone with respect. Remember that we are dependent on each other just as lions are dependent on grass.

---

tasks:

workout: none
- ☐ rest

cardio: none
- ☐ rest

nutrition:
- ☐ drink at least eight 8-ounce cups of water
- ☐ take a multivitamin
- ☐ eat only lean meats, fish, seafood, nuts, fruits and vegetables
- ☐ drink 1 serving of a protein shake before breakfast and dinner
- ☐ enjoy sugars, juice, sweets and soda in moderation
- ☐ avoid all artificially colored and processed foods

Sheg Aranmolate, MD

day twenty - nine:
harsh words

> For me, words are a form of action, capable of influencing change.
> Ingrid Bengis

During my sophomore year in college, I decided that I wanted to obtain a second degree in psychology, and to do so I needed to take several psychology courses, one of which was abnormal psychology. In this class, I got to watch several informational videos which discussed the fragility and vulnerability of the human mind. I remember watching a touching documentary about a group of women who were living with or recovering from severe eating disorders. It was sad to watch as many of these beautiful women said that their disorders began when someone, usually a loved one, had verbally abused them or had called them fat. For me, this confirmed that our words are powerful enough to physically and psychologically hurt others. Many of us are often oblivious of the power and irreparable damage that our words can inflict on others. Simply put, our mouths can be like loaded guns with bullets made of words, and just as guns can misfire if incorrectly handled, careless mouths can also misfire. For this reason, we must be careful of what we say and how and when we say it because our words could misfire and severely hurt our loved ones. In the future, when you are 'pissed-off" and want to say hurtful words to someone else, take a moment to think about the possible psychological effects that could result from those words. Remember that once those words are out of your mouth, they can never be retrieved or taken back. Be careful! You never know when your words might be the difference between a happy person and a broken one.

workout: chest

☐ incline bench press   [10 reps x 5 times]

weights (lbs):					

☐ decline bench press   [10 reps x 5 times]

weights (lbs):					

☐ flat bench press   [10 reps x 5 times]

weights (lbs):					

☐ pec deck   [10 reps x 5 times]

weights (lbs):					

☐ hammer press   [10 reps x 5 times]

weights (lbs):					

☐ dips   [20 reps x 5 times]

weights (lbs):					

cardio: treadmill

☐ paced walk/jog   [30 minutes]

calories:	

nutrition:

☐ drink at least eight 8-ounce cups of water
☐ take a multivitamin
☐ eat only lean meats, fish, seafood, nuts, fruits and vegetables
☐ drink 1 serving of a protein shake before breakfast and dinner
☐ avoid starches, grains, sugars, juice, sweets and soda
☐ avoid all artificially colored and processed foods

day thirty:
fight it

Choose the life that is most useful, and habit will make it the most agreeable.

Sir Francis Bacon

Toddlers are adorable and curious little beings, and many of them, at the slightest opportunity, will place any object, edible or poisonous, into their mouths. Any responsible parent will tell you that they're always looking for dangerous objects that their child might try swallowing. As a result, any reasonable guardian should know that it is unwise to leave an opened bottle of colorful prescription pills close to a toddler as the child will likely consume the medications. Many of us as adults, although we will not want to compare ourselves to toddlers, act and behave like toddlers especially when it comes to managing our addictions. It's quite obvious that different people have different vices, some of which are socially acceptable and others socially repulsive. Nevertheless, if your addiction is harmful to your health and is ruining your relationship with your loved ones, then you have to ditch that habit-- keep yourself away from it! Many of us, like toddlers, are unable to control ourselves in the presence of our addictive substances. For example, people trying to quit smoking find it hard to resist cigarettes when amongst people who are smoking. Our difficulty in resisting temptations isn't because we're losers, rather it's because of our flawed biological makeup. On the other hand, we need to become more responsible (like parents of toddlers), and continually remove toxic and addictive substances from our vicinity. For instance, if you're trying to quit smoking or junk food, never buy or stock your homes with these things. Keeping your eyes and mind away from addictive substances can help you prevent a relapse. When it comes to addictions, always remember that 'out of sight is out of mind."

workout: back/traps

☐ deadlift   [10 reps x 5 times]

weights (lbs):					

☐ pulldowns   [10 reps x 5 times]

weights (lbs):					

☐ bent over row   [10 reps x 5 times]

weights (lbs):					

☐ cable row   [10 reps x 5 times]

weights (lbs):					

☐ pull ups   [10 reps x 5 times]

weights (lbs):					

☐ shrugs   [10 reps x 5 times]

weights (lbs):					

cardio: stairmaster

☐ paced walk   [30 minutes]

calories:	

nutrition:

☐ drink at least eight 8-ounce cups of water
☐ take a multivitamin
☐ eat only lean meats, fish, seafood, nuts, fruits and vegetables
☐ drink 1 serving of a protein shake before breakfast and dinner
☐ avoid starches, grains, sugars, juice, sweets and soda
☐ avoid all artificially colored and processed foods

day thirty - one:
<u>finding happy</u>

> The pursuit of happiness is a most ridiculous phrase; if you
> pursue happiness you'll never find it.
> <u>C. P. Snow</u>

I was once window-shopping in front of an upscale jewelry store that sold expensive stones. While I was glancing at the dazzling offerings, I noticed two women in the store. The first woman wasn't wearing jewelry and was neatly dressed in casual clothes, while the other woman, in stark contrast, wore a huge, expensive looking necklace and designer clothes. As I continued window-shopping, I immediately concluded that the woman in the expensive clothes was rich and the other woman in the causal clothes was simply window-shopping, like myself. To my surprise, it turned out that the woman in the casual clothes was the owner of the store, inspecting her merchandise; the woman in the designer clothes was in fact the customer. We tend to make assumptions solely based on what we see. For instance, when we see people who are nicely dressed or wearing expensive items, we right away assume that they are financially successful and happy. The truth, however, is that looks can be deceiving as all that glitters is neither platinum nor gold. Over the years, I have come to realize that a large number of wealthy people who are happy with life tend to have relatively normal lives and average lifestyles. I suppose this is because they know that extravagance or excessive spending doesn't always bring happiness. Please don't be misled by a person's outward appearance alone because there are lots of financially successful people who are emotionally destitute, begging and searching for the slightest signs of joy and happiness. Save yourself the heartache and realize that if you're never happy with just enough, you can't be happy with more.

tasks:

workout: legs

☐ squats   [10 reps x 5 times]

weights (lbs):				

☐ squat to bench   [10 reps x 5 times]

weights (lbs):				

☐ quad extensions   [15 reps x 5 times]

weights (lbs):				

☐ leg curls   [15 reps x 5 times]

weights (lbs):				

☐ leg press calf raises   [20 reps x 5 times]

weights (lbs):				

☐ seated calf raises   [20 reps x 5 times]

weights (lbs):				

cardio: elliptical

☐ paced walk   [30 minutes]

calories:	

nutrition:

☐ drink at least eight 8-ounce cups of water
☐ take a multivitamin
☐ eat only lean meats, fish, seafood, nuts, fruits and vegetables
☐ drink 1 serving of a protein shake before breakfast and dinner
☐ avoid starches, grains, sugars, juice, sweets and soda
☐ avoid all artificially colored and processed foods

day thirty - two:
rock bottom

> Nothing fails like success.
> Gerald Nachman

There are times in our lives when we become unhappy, feeling like our lives have reached rock-bottom. Such miserable times are often the effects of drastic changes in our lives, such as the loss of or estrangement from a loved one, health problems, financial difficulties or sometimes no apparent reason. Regardless of the cause or reason, the truth is that these moments make us feel worthless, like our entire world has hopelessly crashed down. If we took a closer look at our situation, however, we will usually realize that we can use the rock-bottom feeling as an incentive to improve and turn around our lives. Rock-bottom is the lowest possible point that we could find ourselves and because our lives can't get any worse, it can be a unique opportunity for us to reevaluate the composition of our foundation and rebuild our lives for the better. For example, if a rock-climber rapidly ascends up a mountain, but due to inexperience with the route, grabs onto a loose rock and falls to the bottom (literally rock-bottom!), then, during the next climb, this climber will know how to avoid such a pratfall. Do you feel full of despair or like you've reached rock-bottom? It is easier said than done but remember that rock-bottom can be a grand opportunity to start afresh and set things right. Please don't let sorrows or setbacks get the best of you and deprive you of your true glorious potential. Instead, garner all your strength along with all your previously acquired knowledge and climb higher than you have ever before!

tasks:

workout: deltoids

☐ military press behind the neck   [10 reps x 5 times]

weights (lbs):					

☐ military press   [10 reps x 5 times]

weights (lbs):					

☐ dumbbell shoulder press   [10 reps x 5 times]

weights (lbs):					

☐ machine shoulder press   [10 reps x 5 times]

weights (lbs):					

☐ reverse pec deck   [10 reps x 5 times]

weights (lbs):					

☐ dumbbell front raises   [20 reps x 5 times]

weights (lbs):					

cardio: treadmill

☐ paced walk/jog   [30 minutes]

calories:	

nutrition:

☐ drink at least eight 8-ounce cups of water
☐ take a multivitamin
☐ eat only lean meats, fish, seafood, nuts, fruits and vegetables
☐ drink 1 serving of a protein shake before breakfast and dinner
☐ avoid starches, grains, sugars, juice, sweets and soda
☐ avoid all artificially colored and processed foods

day thirty - three:
fashion style

> People grow through experience if they meet life honestly
> and courageously. This is how character is built.
> <u>Eleanor Roosevelt</u>

When we wake up each morning, we usually have a daily routine, including brushing our teeth, taking a shower and drinking coffee. Still, there comes a point when we have to decide what clothes to wear and usually turn to the weather forecast for guidance. It is undeniable that we primarily wear clothes to cover our nakedness and to protect us from the elements of nature such as the heat, the cold and insects. But we also wear clothes for special occasions and to show off social status or our sense of style. It is unfortunate that many of us have become engulfed and enslaved by this need to display. We have become so concerned with our appearance that we allow our feelings to be governed by what we wear. For instance, I have met several people who become unhappy if they feel their clothes aren't fashionable enough. To save some heartache and reduce stress, we need to stop worrying excessively about our clothes because they fade and rip with time. Rather, we should start focusing on our 'emotional clothes," i.e. the positive emotions we show other people. If there was a way to judge people by their emotional clothes, it may come as no surprise that some of us are poorly dressed in rags of anger, despair and even hatred. Please take the time today to clean out your emotional closet of those raggedy clothes and replace them with clothes of kindness, compassion, altruism and honesty. People will definitely appreciate and some might even envy your new emotional style.

tasks:

workout: arms/forearms

☐ pushdowns   [10 reps x 5 times]

weights (lbs):					

☐ wide grip curls   [10 reps x 5 times]

weights (lbs):					

☐ single arm cable kickbacks   [10 reps x 5 times]

weights (lbs):					

☐ seated triceps press   [10 reps x 5 times]

weights (lbs):					

☐ hammer curls   [10 reps x 5 times]

weights (lbs):					

☐ concentration curls   [20 reps x 5 times]

weights (lbs):					

cardio: stairmaster

☐ paced walk   [30 minutes]

calories:	

nutrition:

☐ drink at least eight 8-ounce cups of water
☐ take a multivitamin
☐ eat only lean meats, fish, seafood, nuts, fruits and vegetables
☐ drink 1 serving of a protein shake before breakfast and dinner
☐ avoid starches, grains, sugars, juice, sweets and soda
☐ avoid all artificially colored and processed foods

Sheg Aranmolate, MD

day thirty - four:
dynamic change

> Never confuse movement with action.
> Ernest Hemingway

Suppose that one day, while you are watching your favorite TV show, a commercial for a charitable organization begins, pleading for funds to feed a bunch of starving children with protruding bellies. These types of commercials usually make us sad because humans are generally kind-hearted and hate to see others suffer. After the commercial, a number of us will probably complain about all the injustice and greed in the world and further conclude that those starving kids will be better off if more rich people gave to the poor. The truth, however, is that many of us, in our rants against the rich, fail to identify our own greed and inadequacy. Wealth is relative. For instance, a millionaire is poorer than a billionaire, but to a person with only a few pennies, both people are extremely rich. If we are to be honest with ourselves, many of us have enough money and resources to help the needy, but because of our excuses or rationalizations we usually end up doing nothing. We're like broken cell phones that are capable of receiving incoming calls but incapable of making outgoing calls. Everyday, we receive so much information on the suffering of others, yet we do nothing to change the world. In fact, in an ironic manner, these disheartening issues sometimes become the latest gossip amongst those people who actually care about the news. Change in our society requires consciously taking action, and every one of us has the ability to produce positive change. Next time please don't just complain about other people's inaction and those issues that affect your families, friends and humanity; try to do something to help out. Remember that actions always speak louder than words, and words always speak louder than absolute silence.

tasks:

workout: abs/core

☐ weighted sit ups   [20 reps x 5 times]

weights (lbs):					

☐ weighted cable crunch   [10 reps x 5 times]

weights (lbs):					

☐ leg raises   [20 reps x 5 times]

weights (lbs):					

☐ air bike   [60 reps x 5 times]

weights (lbs):					

☐ side bends   [40 reps x 5 times]

weights (lbs):					

☐ hanging leg raises   [20 reps x 5 times]

weights (lbs):					

cardio: elliptical

☐ paced walk   [30 minutes]

calories:	

nutrition:

☐ drink at least eight 8-ounce cups of water
☐ take a multivitamin
☐ eat only lean meats, fish, seafood, nuts, fruits and vegetables
☐ drink 1 serving of a protein shake before breakfast and dinner
☐ avoid starches, grains, sugars, juice, sweets and soda
☐ avoid all artificially colored and processed foods

Sheg Aranmolate, MD

day thirty - five:
steady moves

> You can't wait for inspiration. You have to go after it with a club.
>
> Jack London

I once tutored children in elementary and middle school. On my first day with the kids, in order to gauge their perception of the world, I always ask them what they wanted to do as adults. Many of the kids had great choices such as lawyers, doctors, teachers and police officers to name a few. I was often amazed that kids are so conscious of the world around them and harbor great desires to make it better. As a result, it is quite disheartening that as they become older and are subjected to harsh realities in the world, some of their amazing plans never get executed or accomplished. The same occurs with the dreams of some adults like ending world starvation and curing human diseases. Many of us never get to fulfill our dreams not because we are procrastinators--actually maybe we are slight procrastinators! On a more serious note, the truth is that we live in a world filled with responsibilities. We are consumed with caring for our families and paying our bills that we consequently have little time to execute our great ideas. Nonetheless, our responsibilities shouldn't be a reason for us to forgo all our dreams, rather they should an incentive for us to complete them. The truth is that no matter how much resources you have or do not have at your disposal, you can't build your dream home overnight, just as you can't change the entire world in one night. However, by taking a few minutes out of each day you can pursue parts of your dreams. If you're genuinely keen on making a difference in the world, you can start by improving yourself, then your family, your community and finally the entire world. Remember that the great pyramids of Giza were built block by block.

tasks:

workout: none
☐ rest

cardio: none
☐ rest

nutrition:
☐ drink at least eight 8-ounce cups of water
☐ take a multivitamin
☐ eat only lean meats, fish, seafood, nuts, fruits and vegetables
☐ drink 1 serving of a protein shake before breakfast and dinner
☐ enjoy sugars, juice, sweets and soda in moderation
☐ avoid all artificially colored and processed foods

Sheg Aranmolate, MD

day thirty – six:
reconstruction

A good name, like good will, is got by many actions and lost
by one.
Lord Jeffery

Recently, I visited my old college to see old friends and professors, and was amazed by how much the campus, in only a few years, had changed. Several new buildings had been erected and there were other construction projects in progress. I noticed that the students and many new professors seemed much younger than when I was there. I suddenly came to the realization that I was getting older and my beloved college had changed without me. Change, after all, is a part of life and we are always changing our environment through continual planned demolition and construction projects. For instance, we demolish old bridges so we can construct, stronger, better bridges. Old buildings are converted to skyscrapers and the list continues. Our lives can be similar to a construction project. Sometimes we learn new facts and experience new situations that require us to demolish and reconstruct our views and perspectives of the world. Often, these newly-formed ideas are stronger than the older ones. If you are familiar with construction, then you know it can take several years to build a large building like a skyscraper or cathedral, but only a few seconds to destroy it. Similarly, many of us also take years to construct our architecturally sound lives, but demolish them with one simple mistake. Remember that we live in a world that requires change and no matter how wonderful your life may seem one slipup can cost you everything. Always be patient in forming your ideas, please don't be afraid to reconstruct them if you are wrong and avoid those destructive elements that can ruin your life. Nevertheless, with time and patience you can always rebuild your life, no matter how bad you may have 'ruined" it.

---

workout: chest

☐ incline bench press [10 reps x 5 times]

weights (lbs):					

☐ decline bench press [10 reps x 5 times]

weights (lbs):					

☐ flat bench press [10 reps x 5 times]

weights (lbs):					

☐ pec deck [10 reps x 5 times]

weights (lbs):					

☐ hammer press [10 reps x 5 times]

weights (lbs):					

☐ dips [20 reps x 5 times]

weights (lbs):					

cardio: treadmill

☐ paced walk/jog [30 minutes]

calories:	

nutrition:

☐ drink at least eight 8-ounce cups of water
☐ take a multivitamin
☐ eat only lean meats, fish, seafood, nuts, fruits and vegetables
☐ drink 1 serving of a protein shake before breakfast and dinner
☐ avoid starches, grains, sugars, juice, sweets and soda
☐ avoid all artificially colored and processed foods

Sheg Aranmolate, MD

day thirty - seven:
active gestures

> Never doubt that a small group of thoughtful, committed citizens can change the world. Indeed, it is the only thing that ever has.
> Margaret Mead

If you have ever walked on the busy streets of one of the many developing nations, then surely you've encountered malnourished children, begging desperately for food or some money. It is quite sad but due to the multitude of these kids on the streets, many of their cries and pleas are often shunned by stoic pedestrians. Every now and then, a passing adult still get touched by the children's plight and will stop to offer them food or money. Over time many of these initially compassionate adults also become callous to the suffering of these children. This is not because they are all terrible people, rather because they join the masses and accept defeat, concluding that the suffering of these kids is a normal part of their society. All humans, by default and by the characterization as being 'human," are equal, and there shouldn't be any reason, why one person should enjoy and another should suffer things like starvation and terrible living conditions. How will you like to be one of those orphans starving daily, only to hear adults conclude that your pain is a normal part of society? It's undeniable that we live in a world filled with much pain and suffering. Many of us are still fortunate enough and have the ability to make a positive difference in our unjust world. Remember that the entire world is our home, and just as we can't leave all the maintenance, service and chores to one parent or sibling, we can't leave the eradication of the world's problems to one nation, organization or person. Instead, we should all take active roles in our communities and society to ensure that we minimize the suffering of other people.

tasks:

workout: back/traps

☐ deadlift   [10 reps x 5 times]

weights (lbs):					

☐ pulldowns   [10 reps x 5 times]

weights (lbs):					

☐ bent over row   [10 reps x 5 times]

weights (lbs):					

☐ cable row   [10 reps x 5 times]

weights (lbs):					

☐ pull ups   [10 reps x 5 times]

weights (lbs):					

☐ shrugs   [10 reps x 5 times]

weights (lbs):					

cardio: stairmaster

☐ paced walk   [30 minutes]

calories:	

nutrition:

☐ drink at least eight 8-ounce cups of water
☐ take a multivitamin
☐ eat only lean meats, fish, seafood, nuts, fruits and vegetables
☐ drink 1 serving of a protein shake before breakfast and dinner
☐ avoid starches, grains, sugars, juice, sweets and soda
☐ avoid all artificially colored and processed foods

Sheg Aranmolate, MD

day thirty - eight:
blissful manners

> The greatest griefs are those we cause ourselves.
> <u>Sophocles</u>

Happiness and sadness are two common emotions, and beginning in childhood society teaches us that it is good to be happy and bad to be sad. It is expected that we become happy when we hear good news and saddened when we hear bad news. As a result, we are all quite familiar with the tingling feel-good sensation of happiness and the burning sensation of sadness. Despite these disparate sensations of happiness and sadness, many of us, in a matter of seconds, can quickly switch from being happy to being sad, but can't quickly switch from being sad to being happy. One minute we're happy and the very next minute we can feel like we've never experienced happiness in our lives. Why don't we feel sad when we hear good news and happy when we hear bad news? In theory, it's possible because our 'defined" emotions, such as happiness, sadness, love, hate or anger are the combination of certain feelings attached to words. Technically and philosophically, the feelings of happiness or sadness in one person can be very different in another person. For this reason, many of us might not happy perhaps because we are living in prisons constructed by our limited definitions of our emotions. Please don't limit your sense of happiness to what you think defines happiness! Set yourself free, and realize that there are several other feelings and ideas that encompass idle happiness. But because of our limited definitions, many of us unwisely never consider these feelings and ideas as reasons to be happy. Happiness, like beauty, is defined by the beholder and because we are the beholders, we should strive to behold ourselves as happy.

tasks:

workout: legs

☐ squats   [10 reps x 5 times]

weights (lbs):			

☐ squat to bench   [10 reps x 5 times]

weights (lbs):			

☐ quad extensions   [15 reps x 5 times]

weights (lbs):			

☐ leg curls   [15 reps x 5 times]

weights (lbs):			

☐ leg press calf raises   [20 reps x 5 times]

weights (lbs):			

☐ seated calf raises   [20 reps x 5 times]

weights (lbs):			

cardio: elliptical

☐ paced walk   [30 minutes]

calories:

nutrition:

☐ drink at least eight 8-ounce cups of water
☐ take a multivitamin
☐ eat only lean meats, fish, seafood, nuts, fruits and vegetables
☐ drink 1 serving of a protein shake before breakfast and dinner
☐ avoid starches, grains, sugars, juice, sweets and soda
☐ avoid all artificially colored and processed foods

Sheg Aranmolate, MD

day thirty - nine:
a cruel world

> I finally realized that being grateful to my body was key to
> giving more love to myself.
> <u>Oprah Winfrey</u>

When I was about eight years old in Nigeria, I was driving with my father, a reconstructive surgeon, in heavy traffic. A young man with lots of scar tissue and contracture from burns suddenly approached us, begging for money. Instead of giving him money, my father gave him his business card and offered to help him secure free surgical treatment for his burns. To my surprise, I later learned that the man had followed up and politely refused my father's offer. He said that ever since he got burned and started begging, he was making more money to feed his family than he did before his accident, when he worked long grueling hours as an unskilled laborer. As a young boy I failed to understand this man's response, but several years later I came to realize his honesty in light of some of the injustice in our world. Every time I think about this man with his extreme facial disfiguration and his refusal to get surgical treatment, I become upset with the blatant corruption and injustice in several parts of the world. These thoughts and feelings, however, make me extremely grateful for my own life. Nowadays, I try not to complain and take things for granted because I know for a fact that my life could be much worse, just like the millions of people around the world trapped in unfortunate circumstances. It is a little disheartening though that many of us with comfortable lives are quick to complain about petty things. Next time you're about to complain unnecessarily, please take a few moments to think about all the people like the burnt man who would love to be in your current position. There are far more important things in life for anyone to be bogged down with the petty stuff. Live every moment with appreciation for life itself.

---

workout: deltoids

☐ military press behind the neck   [10 reps x 5 times]

weights (lbs):					

☐ military press   [10 reps x 5 times]

weights (lbs):					

☐ dumbbell shoulder press   [10 reps x 5 times]

weights (lbs):					

☐ machine shoulder press   [10 reps x 5 times]

weights (lbs):					

☐ reverse pec deck   [10 reps x 5 times]

weights (lbs):					

☐ dumbbell front raises   [20 reps x 5 times]

weights (lbs):					

cardio: treadmill

☐ paced walk/jog   [30 minutes]

calories:	

nutrition:

☐ drink at least eight 8-ounce cups of water
☐ take a multivitamin
☐ eat only lean meats, fish, seafood, nuts, fruits and vegetables
☐ drink 1 serving of a protein shake before breakfast and dinner
☐ avoid starches, grains, sugars, juice, sweets and soda
☐ avoid all artificially colored and processed foods

day forty:
the right attitude

> Human beings, by changing the inner attitudes of their
> minds, can change the outer aspects of their lives.
> <u>William James</u>

I define attitude or an attitude as a person's feelings towards any particular aspect of his or her life, and it should come as no surprise that our attitudes affect the world. Our attitudes surround us like an aura, and are capable of directly and indirectly influencing our activities and those of others. Therefore, someone with a positive attitude usually acts in a positive manner and positively influences other people, while a negative person gives off negative energy. Nevertheless, I still find it strange that many of us seem forgetful or oblivious to this fact and take our attitudes towards life and towards others for granted. Children, because of their innocence and sincerity, demonstrate the importance of our attitudes. If you watch a group of children playing, you will notice that their displayed attitude towards each other affects the overall dynamics of the playground. For example, a child with a positive attitude will likely play well with others, but a child with a negative attitude will likely start fights with others. It is amazing that one sullen child in a playground can project his or her attitude onto other kids, making them all sullen as well. Have you ever seen a group of kids playing together, when suddenly one child starts to cry and the others begin to cry as well? Well, that's the power of attitude on behavior! A truly positive attitude towards life is the foundation to maintaining a happy life. Please always remember to be positive because positive people are happier and usually more successful than negative people.

---

workout: arms/forearms

☐ pushdowns   [10 reps x 5 times]

weights (lbs):					

☐ wide grip curls   [10 reps x 5 times]

weights (lbs):					

☐ single arm cable kickbacks   [10 reps x 5 times]

weights (lbs):					

☐ seated triceps press   [10 reps x 5 times]

weights (lbs):					

☐ hammer curls   [10 reps x 5 times]

weights (lbs):					

☐ concentration curls   [20 reps x 5 times]

weights (lbs):					

cardio: stairmaster

☐ paced walk   [30 minutes]

calories:	

nutrition:

☐ drink at least eight 8-ounce cups of water
☐ take a multivitamin
☐ eat only lean meats, fish, seafood, nuts, fruits and vegetables
☐ drink 1 serving of a protein shake before breakfast and dinner
☐ avoid starches, grains, sugars, juice, sweets and soda
☐ avoid all artificially colored and processed foods

day forty - one:
added effort

> Energy and persistence conquer all things.
> <u>Benjamin Franklin</u>

As a fitness trainer, I often received letters from people who wanted the secret to getting into shape and losing weight without exercise. I frankly told them that no such secret exists, and that they should ignore diet programs and pills claiming to be the easy answer. For many of us, getting into shape, like several aspects of our lives, can be more like running a marathon than running a short sprint. If you've ever trained for a marathon, then you know how much focus and endurance that marathons demand. Also, you know that there are times when you want to quit, not because you are a coward, rather because of the grueling nature of a long run. There are days when life gets tough and we want to quit on ourselves. However, just like long days at work, we must meet the challenge and keep trying. This 'never-giving-up" attitude is required to tackle those days when we are confronted with life's challenges. Interestingly, our fast paced lifestyles and our desire for instant gratification are often the biggest reasons why many of us fail some of life's challenges. We have forgotten that certain aspects of life require patience and large amounts of time to mature. Come on, let's be honest with ourselves. You can't pop a pill, eat whatever you like and then go to sleep flabby, expecting to wake up with bulging biceps and washboard abs. Just like acquiring a new language or learning a new subject in mathematics, fitness requires time and sustained effort. Please don't be fooled into thinking you can meet life's challenges with a pill and without the necessary time and effort.

workout: abs/core

☐ weighted sit ups   [20 reps x 5 times]

weights (lbs):					

☐ weighted cable crunch   [10 reps x 5 times]

weights (lbs):					

☐ leg raises   [20 reps x 5 times]

weights (lbs):					

☐ air bike   [60 reps x 5 times]

weights (lbs):					

☐ side bends   [40 reps x 5 times]

weights (lbs):					

☐ hanging leg raises   [20 reps x 5 times]

weights (lbs):					

cardio: elliptical

☐ paced walk   [30 minutes]

calories:	

nutrition:

☐ drink at least eight 8-ounce cups of water
☐ take a multivitamin
☐ eat only lean meats, fish, seafood, nuts, fruits and vegetables
☐ drink 1 serving of a protein shake before breakfast and dinner
☐ avoid starches, grains, sugars, juice, sweets and soda
☐ avoid all artificially colored and processed foods

day forty - two:
flat tires

The only thing that overcomes hard luck is hard work.
Harry Golden (1902 - 1981)

The road to success is like driving on the highway from one town to another. Consequently, many of the rules of the road can be applied to our lives. For example, just like cars on the highway get stalled in traffic at rush-hour, many of us also get stalled at certain points of our lives by several factors that are beyond our control. However, during those times it is important that we remain steadfast and persevere until the road becomes clear. Over the years, I have heard people complain about how hard it is to succeed in life, and how the ideas of endurance and perseverance are overrated. It is true that life can get tough and perseverance or endurance can be far from easy, but with the appropriate mindset many of the tough aspects of life can be easier to approach. Perseverance without motivation is similar to driving a car with flat tires. Any driver should know that flat tires on a car need to be corrected before the car is driven because the consequences of doing otherwise can be dangerous. Likewise, in order for us to persevere through those tough times in life, we need good 'motivational tires" to keep us focused and ensure that we don't get stalled during our journey in life. For this reason, it is important that we surround ourselves with good people and positive ideas that continuously motivate and help us strive to the end. Please don't be irrational and drive your life on flat tires. If you are stressed out and feel like you're unable to continue your strive through life, it might be a true indicator that you need to take some time off to repair and refill your 'motivational tires," so that you don't get involved in a tragic accident in life.

workout: none
☐ rest

cardio: none
☐ rest

nutrition:
☐ drink at least eight 8-ounce cups of water
☐ take a multivitamin
☐ eat only lean meats, fish, seafood, nuts, fruits and vegetables
☐ drink 1 serving of a protein shake before breakfast and dinner
☐ enjoy sugars, juice, sweets and soda in moderation
☐ avoid all artificially colored and processed foods

day forty - three:
the blueprint

> A goal without a plan is just a wish.
> Antoine de Saint-Exupery

For many simple things in life, we have a plan or plans for doing them. For instance, we go to the grocery store with the plan to buy groceries and to the mechanic to get our car fixed. Many of us know from experience that having goals without the plans to achieve them usually results in failure. For example, if you impulsively walked into the kitchen without a recipe and randomly mixed several foods together into a dish (e.g. bananas, peas, vinegar, tomatoes and sauerkraut), it's unlikely that the dish will be good. It is even more unlikely that you will produce a gourmet dish because gourmet dishes, like many aspects of our lives, require appropriate planning. Many of us at times become frustrated with how disorganized we are in achieving our goals. We, however, fail to realize that our lack of plans for the future is the main reason for our woes. Please let's be honest with ourselves! How can we ever set things right, if we can't distinguish our left from our right? An important key to becoming successful in life is to set reasonable goals with multiple plans (i.e. plan A, plan B, etc.). It's also crucial that we take time out of our chaotic lives to write down the brilliant plans and goals that we want accomplished. This forces us to think about our true desires, but it also sets our creative minds and thoughts into motion to help us achieve our desires. It is important to remember that no one, no matter how talented, resourceful or gifted, can build an architecturally sound skyscraper, house or bridge without a detailed and meticulously designed blueprint. Today, make plans to achieve all your future goals of tomorrow.

---

tasks:

workout: chest

☐ incline bench press   [10 reps x 5 times]

weights (lbs):					

☐ decline bench press   [10 reps x 5 times]

weights (lbs):					

☐ flat bench press   [10 reps x 5 times]

weights (lbs):					

☐ pec deck   [10 reps x 5 times]

weights (lbs):					

☐ hammer press   [10 reps x 5 times]

weights (lbs):					

☐ dips   [20 reps x 5 times]

weights (lbs):					

cardio: treadmill

☐ paced walk/jog   [30 minutes]

calories:	

nutrition:

☐ drink at least eight 8-ounce cups of water
☐ take a multivitamin
☐ eat only lean meats, fish, seafood, nuts, fruits and vegetables
☐ drink 1 serving of a protein shake before breakfast and dinner
☐ avoid starches, grains, sugars, juice, sweets and soda
☐ avoid all artificially colored and processed foods

day forty - four:
the privileged ones

> The only thing to do with good advice is pass it on. It is never
> any use to oneself.
>
> Oscar Wilde

Have you ever taken time out of your busy life to appreciate all the wonderful things around you? If you have, then you know that regardless of all the turmoil in the world there is still much love and affection. If you have not, then are missing out. The ability to reflect is unique to humans, and it's unfortunate that many of us don't seem to use this gift to free ourselves from the stresses of life. Once, I was watching a TV show about people addicted to drugs, and many addicts said that they began using drugs to alleviate their stress. It will be ignorant for anyone to assume that we don't live in a stressful world, but abusing drugs is definitely not the way out. Nevertheless, I hope such people can eventually turn to self-reflection as a way to break their addictions and alleviate stress. Abusing drugs is similar to placing a bandage over an injury that requires immediate surgery, and if you're familiar with medicine, then you should know that a bandage alone will not do the trick. A good way to start harnessing the power of reflection is to think about how blessed you are to simply be alive, especially given all the diseases and other dangers in the world. Think of people in developing or war-torn countries or those who suffer illnesses like cancer or AIDS. This should really put your blessings in perspective and at least alleviate some stress. It is quite intriguing and perhaps ironic that the ability for many people to abuse expensive drugs is actually a privilege and a luxury. Please remember that your very existence is a cause for celebration and you should let other people know this fact. Be nice and compassionate to everyone and you will see that there is so much happiness inside of you.

workout: back/traps

☐ deadlift   [10 reps x 5 times]

weights (lbs):					

☐ pulldowns   [10 reps x 5 times]

weights (lbs):					

☐ bent over row   [10 reps x 5 times]

weights (lbs):					

☐ cable row   [10 reps x 5 times]

weights (lbs):					

☐ pull ups   [10 reps x 5 times]

weights (lbs):					

☐ shrugs   [10 reps x 5 times]

weights (lbs):					

cardio: stairmaster

☐ paced walk   [30 minutes]

calories:	

nutrition:

☐ drink at least eight 8-ounce cups of water
☐ take a multivitamin
☐ eat only lean meats, fish, seafood, nuts, fruits and vegetables
☐ drink 1 serving of a protein shake before breakfast and dinner
☐ avoid starches, grains, sugars, juice, sweets and soda
☐ avoid all artificially colored and processed foods

day forty - five:
beauty standards

> The absence of flaw in beauty is itself a flaw.
>
Havelock Ellis

I t's always heartbreaking to hear beautiful people with so much potential call themselves ugly and worthless. Time and time again, I try to understand why some people mistreat themselves this way. There is no doubt that we live in an image-conscious society, where people use certain standards and requirements to define beauty. However, because we are human, the truth is that everyone is beautiful, regardless of height, weight, race or any other characteristic. The words 'human" and 'being" encompasses so much beauty that it's absurd some of us constantly subject ourselves to ridiculous standards of beauty. The ideas of beauty and ugliness are emotional states of mind. For instance, it's very likely that the last time you were angry and happened to look in the mirror, you didn't feel beautiful. It's equally possible that the last time someone complimented you on, say, your hair, you did feel so. But we should not let our emotions determine our sense of beauty. We should break free and appreciate all the beauty emanating from inside us and others. In all honestly, why does anyone want to be like the norm? The truth is that if everyone on earth looked like the 'perfect" models in the magazine, the world will be a very boring place and there will probably be new standards of beauty. This, however, doesn't mean that we should not maintain a healthy weight or care for our bodies through proper diet and adequate exercise. Please take a walk around your neighborhood and observe the beauty of diversity in people. People say that beauty is in the eye of the beholder, so when you look in the mirror, behold yourself as beautiful.

---

tasks:

workout: legs

☐ squats   [10 reps x 5 times]

weights (lbs):				

☐ squat to bench   [10 reps x 5 times]

weights (lbs):				

☐ quad extensions   [15 reps x 5 times]

weights (lbs):				

☐ leg curls   [15 reps x 5 times]

weights (lbs):				

☐ leg press calf raises   [20 reps x 5 times]

weights (lbs):				

☐ seated calf raises   [20 reps x 5 times]

weights (lbs):				

cardio: elliptical

☐ paced walk   [30 minutes]

calories:	

nutrition:

☐ drink at least eight 8-ounce cups of water
☐ take a multivitamin
☐ eat only lean meats, fish, seafood, nuts, fruits and vegetables
☐ drink 1 serving of a protein shake before breakfast and dinner
☐ avoid starches, grains, sugars, juice, sweets and soda
☐ avoid all artificially colored and processed foods

Sheg Aranmolate, MD

day forty - six:
diamonds forever

> Courage and perseverance have a magical talisman, before
> which difficulties disappear and obstacles vanish into air.
> John Quincy Adams

Of course, a well-polished diamond has a beautiful luster and shines brilliantly in light. People prize diamonds, so they are very expensive. Many people--especially men--even spend fortunes on diamonds and use them as symbols to show their love and affection towards their significant others. In fact, it has almost become a standard requirement in modern society for engagement and wedding rings to be encrusted with a one or more diamonds. It is quite interesting that many of us are very familiar with the shine of diamonds, but don't know or fully understand the natural formation process of these brilliant and resilient stones. In brief, diamonds are made in nature from carbon, which is usually soft and opaque. Under high heat and pressure, however, the carbon transmutes into hard, brown-hued stones. At this point, diamonds look dull and coarse like any ordinary stone. Only after jewelers cut and polish diamonds do they sparkle. Interestingly, the story of most of our lives is similar to the formation of diamonds. The initial stages of our lives are like the opaque carbon that requires intense heat and pressure to be transformed into diamonds. We must realize that difficult times in our lives, like the time carbon spends under high temperature and pressure, are temporary requirements needed to transform ourselves (our mental, physical and emotional states) from one maturity level to the next. Don't fret during these times as they are worth every resulting carat!

workout: deltoids

☐ military press behind the neck   [10 reps x 5 times]

weights (lbs):					

☐ military press   [10 reps x 5 times]

weights (lbs):					

☐ dumbbell shoulder press   [10 reps x 5 times]

weights (lbs):					

☐ machine shoulder press   [10 reps x 5 times]

weights (lbs):					

☐ reverse pec deck   [10 reps x 5 times]

weights (lbs):					

☐ dumbbell front raises   [20 reps x 5 times]

weights (lbs):					

cardio: treadmill

☐ paced walk/jog   [30 minutes]

calories:	

nutrition:

☐ drink at least eight 8-ounce cups of water
☐ take a multivitamin
☐ eat only lean meats, fish, seafood, nuts, fruits and vegetables
☐ drink 1 serving of a protein shake before breakfast and dinner
☐ avoid starches, grains, sugars, juice, sweets and soda
☐ avoid all artificially colored and processed foods

day forty - seven:
undetectable essence

> While there's life, there's hope.
> Cicero

Obviously, we all live in a physical world! It's therefore easy for us to simply believe in things we can sense with our sensory organs. For instance, many of us follow the 'seeing is believing" ideology: if we can't sense a particular thing, then it simply doesn't exist. This way of thinking is false because there are many things or phenomena in the world that our 'rudimentary" sensory organs cannot detect, such as ultra-violet radiation and radio waves. Over the years, we have learned about their existence and utilize them with the equipment that powers modern life. It is quite important to note that if humans hadn't invented radio receivers to detect the presence of radio waves, technically radio waves wouldn't exist to us. Many of us need to reevaluate our mentality and realize that there are things that exist in the world that we cannot detect with our sensory organs. Presently, there isn't a way to quantitatively measure genuine human emotions and feelings such as patience, kindness, compassion, hatred and even hope or faith. This, however, doesn't disprove the existence and power of emotions. Our emotions and feelings can positively or negatively influence us and others as well, just as invisible magnetic fields can move metallic objects from a distance. Hence, don't wait for physical proofs before you start practicing and showing others genuine positive human emotions such as affection, kindness and compassion. Please don't be blinded with your unawareness, and remember that the inability to measure a human feeling like hope or faith doesn't disprove its existence.

tasks:

workout: arms/forearms

☐ pushdowns   [10 reps x 5 times]

weights (lbs):					

☐ wide grip curls   [10 reps x 5 times]

weights (lbs):					

☐ single arm cable kickbacks   [10 reps x 5 times]

weights (lbs):					

☐ seated triceps press   [10 reps x 5 times]

weights (lbs):					

☐ hammer curls   [10 reps x 5 times]

weights (lbs):					

☐ concentration curls   [20 reps x 5 times]

weights (lbs):					

cardio: stairmaster

☐ paced walk   [30 minutes]

calories:	

nutrition:

☐ drink at least eight 8-ounce cups of water
☐ take a multivitamin
☐ eat only lean meats, fish, seafood, nuts, fruits and vegetables
☐ drink 1 serving of a protein shake before breakfast and dinner
☐ avoid starches, grains, sugars, juice, sweets and soda
☐ avoid all artificially colored and processed foods

day forty - eight:
the laws of time

> Time does not change us. It just unfolds us.
> <u>Max Frisch</u>

I t should come as no surprise that time governs our lives. From the moment we are born to the moment we die, every aspect of our lives evolves around time. For this reason, we are quick to blame time for many of our problems (like when we say 'If only I had enough time"), but fail to acknowledge time for many of our successes. This is similar to the fact that many of us are quick to blame others for our failures in life but are quick to take sole credit for our successes. The amount of time in a given day is constant, and everyone regardless of their creed gets the same amount of time daily. We must realize that we cannot control time (at least not yet!) and we should not take short cuts in life to beat it. In fact, our human capacities govern our interactions with time and like any physical law this cannot be challenged without consequences. We have all probably heard a story about a person who misses being in a fatal car crash by a few seconds because of a red light. If that person was impatient and tried to run the light to save time, then this person will have arrived in time to be involved in the accident. Trying to take such short cuts in life, then, can have very negative consequences. Always be appreciative for every position you find yourself in life, no matter how much 'wasted time" you may feel you accrued in getting there. Realize that such 'wasted time" could have kept you from trouble, like the person saved by the red light.

tasks:

workout: abs/core

☐ weighted sit ups   [20 reps x 5 times]

weights (lbs):					

☐ weighted cable crunch   [10 reps x 5 times]

weights (lbs):					

☐ leg raises   [20 reps x 5 times]

weights (lbs):					

☐ air bike   [60 reps x 5 times]

weights (lbs):					

☐ side bends   [40 reps x 5 times]

weights (lbs):					

☐ hanging leg raises   [20 reps x 5 times]

weights (lbs):					

cardio: elliptical

☐ paced walk   [30 minutes]

calories:	

nutrition:

☐ drink at least eight 8-ounce cups of water
☐ take a multivitamin
☐ eat only lean meats, fish, seafood, nuts, fruits and vegetables
☐ drink 1 serving of a protein shake before breakfast and dinner
☐ avoid starches, grains, sugars, juice, sweets and soda
☐ avoid all artificially colored and processed foods

Sheg Aranmolate, MD

day forty - nine:
ennui

> The cure for boredom is curiosity. There is no cure for
> curiosity.
> <u>Dorothy Parker</u>

Wouldn't it be nice to walk barefoot along the shores of a beautiful beach in the morning? What about horseback riding in the woods with a loved one or eating breakfast on an exotic island? These activities are exciting, but unfortunately many of us don't have the resources or money to do them. Nevertheless, this is no reason why we can't find other exciting things to do in life. No matter who you are or where you live, there are good times to be had. Of course, there will always be times in our lives when things feel monotonous or boring. These feelings, however, are normal because we always long for change. They also surely make the exciting times exciting. We as humans are clearly different from other animals by our unquenchable thirst and desire for change. Consequently, it's not surprising that we often become bored with certain aspects of our lives. The next time you feel bored, however, think about the activities that make you feel alive and then find affordable ways to engage in those activities. For instance, as a child a couple friends and I really liked and enjoyed playing soccer, but at time when we couldn't find soccer balls, we made substitutes out of banana leaves. You might be surprised that a little change or substitution is all you need to get you out of ennui (a state of boredom). But keep in mind that just because an activity makes you feel excited, it doesn't mean that it's good for you. This is because several self-destructive activities might seem exciting at first. Please be smart with your choices, have fun and remember that you don't have to be rich to live an exciting life.

tasks:

workout: none
- ☐ rest

cardio: none
- ☐ rest

nutrition:
- ☐ drink at least eight 8-ounce cups of water
- ☐ take a multivitamin
- ☐ eat only lean meats, fish, seafood, nuts, fruits and vegetables
- ☐ drink 1 serving of a protein shake before breakfast and dinner
- ☐ enjoy sugars, juice, sweets and soda in moderation
- ☐ avoid all artificially colored and processed foods

Sheg Aranmolate, MD

day fifty:
the successful mistake

> Success is the ability to go from one failure to another with
> no loss of enthusiasm.
> <u>Sir Winston Churchill</u>

A few decades ago, if a deep cut on your leg got infected, then you had a high chance of requiring an amputation or dying from shock. However, all this changed with the discovery of Penicillin by Sir Alexander Fleming in 1928. At the time, he was working with some bacteria cultures and realized that a foreign organism had contaminated them. After further experimentation, he discovered that the contaminant--now called Penicillin--was killing the bacteria. Since this lucky discovery, Penicillin has saved millions of lives and is still used today in the fight against many disease-causing bacteria. This story is inspirational because it reveals that sometimes mistakes turn out to be great accomplishments. It is quite unfortunate, however, that many of us may miss these occurrences because society teaches us to like or celebrate our successes, but to dislike or ignore our failures. If Sir Fleming did that, then perhaps people in his time would have missed out on a great discovery. It is also worth noting that our definitions of success and failure are quite subjective! We usually view success as instances when we get 'expected results" and failure as instances when we don't. As a result, many of us continually feel like failures because we expect the 'wrong results" from life and unwisely consider many of our successes as failures. Please be more attentive to your mistakes and try to learn something from them. You never know, your next mistake might actually turn out to be the basis for your greatest achievement in life.

tasks:

workout: chest

☐ incline bench press   [10 reps x 5 times]

weights (lbs):					

☐ decline bench press   [10 reps x 5 times]

weights (lbs):					

☐ flat bench press   [10 reps x 5 times]

weights (lbs):					

☐ pec deck   [10 reps x 5 times]

weights (lbs):					

☐ hammer press   [10 reps x 5 times]

weights (lbs):					

☐ dips   [20 reps x 5 times]

weights (lbs):					

cardio: treadmill

☐ paced walk/jog   [30 minutes]

calories:

nutrition:

☐ drink at least eight 8-ounce cups of water
☐ take a multivitamin
☐ eat only lean meats, fish, seafood, nuts, fruits and vegetables
☐ drink 1 serving of a protein shake before breakfast and dinner
☐ avoid starches, grains, sugars, juice, sweets and soda
☐ avoid all artificially colored and processed foods

Sheg Aranmolate, MD

day fifty - one:
manipulative

> Ninety-nine percent of all failures come from people who
> have the habit of making excuses.
> George Washington Carver

While I was in college, I attended several campus debates. Fellow students would argue about many topics, such as bioethics, politics and pop-culture. These debates were educative and I learned that smart people with the right words can sell a weak point to any audience. During one debate, I remember watching a young man argue his way out of a position that I thought was relatively weak and effortlessly defeat his opponent with his cunning use of the English vocabulary. We all must realize that, just like this young man, we are capable of manipulating words and providing rationalization in defense of negative actions and behaviors. Let's be honest with ourselves: if we are defending a negative behavior or position through rationalization, then we are clearly engaging in deception--self-deception. For example I have heard some people tell me that they are a 'little bit hateful" or a 'little bit hurtful," and as a result they are not hateful or hurtful people. The truth, however, is that positive or negative human behaviors and feelings can't currently be quantified. Therefore, a person can't be a 'little bit" hateful or hurtful. If you have a little bit of hate or a lot of hate, the bottom-line is that you have been hateful. Remember that just as people have different pain thresholds, people also have different emotional thresholds. Hence, what you might consider to be a little bit of hate might be perceived by someone else as the greatest form of hate possible. Please stop the denial and be considerate with your words and actions because like a sharp tool they can be used for good or evil.

tasks:

workout: back/traps

☐ deadlift   [10 reps x 5 times]

weights (lbs):					

☐ pulldowns   [10 reps x 5 times]

weights (lbs):					

☐ bent over row   [10 reps x 5 times]

weights (lbs):					

☐ cable row   [10 reps x 5 times]

weights (lbs):					

☐ pull ups   [10 reps x 5 times]

weights (lbs):					

☐ shrugs   [10 reps x 5 times]

weights (lbs):					

cardio: stairmaster

☐ paced walk   [30 minutes]

calories:	

nutrition:

☐ drink at least eight 8-ounce cups of water
☐ take a multivitamin
☐ eat only lean meats, fish, seafood, nuts, fruits and vegetables
☐ drink 1 serving of a protein shake before breakfast and dinner
☐ avoid starches, grains, sugars, juice, sweets and soda
☐ avoid all artificially colored and processed foods

day fifty - two:
jam-packed

> Do not anticipate trouble, or worry about what may never
> happen. Keep in the sunlight.
> <u>Benjamin Franklin</u>

ave you ever noticed the large amounts of stuff that some people have in their basements and garages? Once, I was helping a family clean out their garage because it was disorganized and could no longer fit a car. As I started cleaning, I discovered that there was a large ratio of junk to valuable items all stacked together, giving it the whole lot a poor appearance. The family's overcrowded garage revealed a unique desire of some humans to continuously acquire and accumulate things. This habit could have dated back to the Stone Ages, when we needed to save things to survive, but who knows? Nevertheless, the truth is that, over time, these acquired items can crowd our lives. Interestingly, our minds--filled with both junk and valuable ideas--can also become like these overstocked garages. Our rubbish ideas, such as thoughts of envy, racism and superiority, can even end up crowding out our many great ideas, making it difficult to access great ideas when we need them. For instance, will you be able to truly help the less-fortunate when your mind is filled thoughts of superiority or racism? Or on a comical note, will you want to discuss serious political or economic issues solely with references to your favorite childhood video game or cartoon character? Always strive for a clean and uncluttered mind so that you don't let those valuable thoughts of yours become overshadowed by worthless and junk ideas. Today, clean out your mind, ditch rubbish ideas and fill your head with good ideas. Please don't be a hoarder and set yourself free from habitual junk collecting!

tasks:

workout: legs

☐ squats   [10 reps x 5 times]

weights (lbs):				

☐ squat to bench   [10 reps x 5 times]

weights (lbs):				

☐ quad extensions   [15 reps x 5 times]

weights (lbs):				

☐ leg curls   [15 reps x 5 times]

weights (lbs):				

☐ leg press calf raises   [20 reps x 5 times]

weights (lbs):				

☐ seated calf raises   [20 reps x 5 times]

weights (lbs):				

cardio: elliptical

☐ paced walk   [30 minutes]

calories:	

nutrition:

☐ drink at least eight 8-ounce cups of water
☐ take a multivitamin
☐ eat only lean meats, fish, seafood, nuts, fruits and vegetables
☐ drink 1 serving of a protein shake before breakfast and dinner
☐ avoid starches, grains, sugars, juice, sweets and soda
☐ avoid all artificially colored and processed foods

Sheg Aranmolate, MD

day fifty - three:
the exaggerator

> The visionary lies to himself, the liar only to others.
> Friedrich Nietzsche

When many people think of great storytellers, they usually think of renowned novelists and authors who have written bestselling books. However, when I think about great storytellers, I think of children. Have you ever heard a child tell a story about a normal event such a trip to the supermarket or a birthday party? If so, then I bet at least parts of the story were beyond belief. Once a boy told me about a birthday party he attended where the cake was bigger than a car. Of course I knew the boy was exaggerating about the huge cake, but not wanting to quell his excitement I played along and acted amazed. Even as adults, there are times when we exaggerate stories for our friends and family. This makes sense, as people often enjoy listening to exaggerations, which make things more engaging and interesting. In story-telling situations, exaggerations can be acceptable distortions of the truth. However, we must realize that exaggerating facts is basically lying. Listeners may therefore come to distrust those who are in the habit of exaggerating stories. If you are a chronic exaggerator, please don't be surprised if others disbelieve your stories or other things you say, even when you are telling the truth. During our everyday lives and when telling stories, it is important to emphasize the most entertaining aspects of the story without exaggerating the truth. Please don't always cry wolf when there are no wolves around because when the wolves truly arrive, no one will be there for the 'exaggerator."

tasks:

workout: deltoids

☐ military press behind the neck   [10 reps x 5 times]

weights (lbs):					

☐ military press   [10 reps x 5 times]

weights (lbs):					

☐ dumbbell shoulder press   [10 reps x 5 times]

weights (lbs):					

☐ machine shoulder press   [10 reps x 5 times]

weights (lbs):					

☐ reverse pec deck   [10 reps x 5 times]

weights (lbs):					

☐ dumbbell front raises   [20 reps x 5 times]

weights (lbs):					

cardio: treadmill

☐ paced walk/jog   [30 minutes]

calories:	

nutrition:

☐ drink at least eight 8-ounce cups of water
☐ take a multivitamin
☐ eat only lean meats, fish, seafood, nuts, fruits and vegetables
☐ drink 1 serving of a protein shake before breakfast and dinner
☐ avoid starches, grains, sugars, juice, sweets and soda
☐ avoid all artificially colored and processed foods

Sheg Aranmolate, MD

day fifty - four:
deceiving looks

> All generalizations are dangerous, even this one.
> Alexandre Dumas

We are all familiar with the saying 'never judge a book by its cover"? Over the years, I have read some great books with terrible covers, and I have also read some terrible books with great covers. We live in an image-conscious world where so many of us tend to make large generalizations based solely on what we observe. This ability to make guesses and generalizations based on what we see might have helped our ancestors survive various poisonous plants and deadly animals, but in current times this ability is no longer so helpful, at least in regards to generalizing people. Honestly, if only many of us took the time to better understand our friends and lovers, rather than being taken by their physical appearance alone, many of us would and could have avoided being involved in hurtful relationships. I am not in any way suggesting that we shouldn't appreciate beauty or beautiful people, but such appreciation should never be the main factor for our choices and decisions. It is quite obvious that it will be ludicrous or unwise for someone to purchase a pretty or sleek-looking car without making sure it has a functional engine. Similarly, why get involved in a relationship without understanding your partner and making sure you are both compatible together? Please be attentive and don't be swindled by appearance alone because to a large extent looks can truly be misleading.

workout: arms/forearms

☐ pushdowns   [10 reps x 5 times]

weights (lbs):					

☐ wide grip curls   [10 reps x 5 times]

weights (lbs):					

☐ single arm cable kickbacks   [10 reps x 5 times]

weights (lbs):					

☐ seated triceps press   [10 reps x 5 times]

weights (lbs):					

☐ hammer curls   [10 reps x 5 times]

weights (lbs):					

☐ concentration curls   [20 reps x 5 times]

weights (lbs):					

cardio: stairmaster

☐ paced walk   [30 minutes]

calories:	

nutrition:

☐ drink at least eight 8-ounce cups of water
☐ take a multivitamin
☐ eat only lean meats, fish, seafood, nuts, fruits and vegetables
☐ drink 1 serving of a protein shake before breakfast and dinner
☐ avoid starches, grains, sugars, juice, sweets and soda
☐ avoid all artificially colored and processed foods

day fifty - five:
the sculptor

> Good judgment comes from experience, and experience
> comes from bad judgment.
> Barry LePatner

If you ever met a person who was saved from drowning by a rescue dog, then it's very likely that this person will be caring towards dogs. In contrast, if this same person was attacked by a dog instead of being rescued, then it's very likely that this person will fear and dislike dogs. It is quite astounding to realize that a lot of our ideas, behaviors and choices are shaped by our various life experiences. Suppose you gave a skilled and an amateur sculptor some clay and told them each to make a statue of an angel: it is likely that the skilled sculptor will do a better job. However, if the skilled sculptor was given dried clay while the amateur was given fresh clay, then it's more likely that the amateur will come out on top. In comparison to our lives, our environments are like the sculptors, capable of shaping us into good or bad angels. A nurturing environment is like a skilled sculptor and a difficult environment is like an amateur sculptor. The difference is that we are not like pieces of clay--we have our own personalities and can get motivated to change, and this can ultimately determine the way our environments shape us. If you are currently in a difficult environment, please don't be discouraged. If you are, then your environment can or might shape you in a negative way against your true destiny. Just think about all the successful people in the world who were once in conditions similar to yours. Always remain tough and steadfast in difficult situations so that you force your environment to shape you in positive ways.

---

tasks:

workout: abs/core

☐ weighted sit ups   [20 reps x 5 times]

weights (lbs):					

☐ weighted cable crunch   [10 reps x 5 times]

weights (lbs):					

☐ leg raises   [20 reps x 5 times]

weights (lbs):					

☐ air bike   [60 reps x 5 times]

weights (lbs):					

☐ side bends   [40 reps x 5 times]

weights (lbs):					

☐ hanging leg raises   [20 reps x 5 times]

weights (lbs):					

cardio: elliptical

☐ paced walk   [30 minutes]

calories:	

nutrition:

☐ drink at least eight 8-ounce cups of water
☐ take a multivitamin
☐ eat only lean meats, fish, seafood, nuts, fruits and vegetables
☐ drink 1 serving of a protein shake before breakfast and dinner
☐ avoid starches, grains, sugars, juice, sweets and soda
☐ avoid all artificially colored and processed foods

Sheg Aranmolate, MD

day fifty - six:
the hiker's pack

> Nothing endures but change.
> Heraclitus

I have gone hiking and jogging in the woods a couple times. For me, hiking is a meditative and invigorating activity that allows my body to exercise and my mind to relax. From experience I can confidently say that having the correct hiking gear is necessary and it can be the difference between having a safe, enjoyable hike or a dangerous and miserable one. There are certain essential items that every camping hiker should have during a hiking trip, such as a good sleeping bag, water bottle, canned food items, utensils and maybe a book or two. However, to make hiking easier it's important to take only essential items because carrying a heavy back-pack can become unbearable after hiking for a few miles. As time goes on while hiking, most backpacks, regardless of how lightly packed, become more of a burden. However, a hiker can't simply throw away his or her pack to lessen the burden because the pack is the hiker's means of survival in the woods. Our journey through life is like hiking. Our everyday obligations, such as our jobs and taking care of family members, are like the essential items in a hiker's back-pack. Similar to how hikers shouldn't toss away their back-packs, we should never desert our jobs or family members. However, when our schedules become too busy and we become overwhelmed with life, it's wise for us to only give up activities that are not essential to our responsibilities and health such as worrying about the latest gossip or obtaining new items or merchandise. Please don't overwhelm yourself with superfluous activities, and instead hold onto the important things in life.

tasks:

workout: none
☐ rest

cardio: none
☐ rest

nutrition:
☐ drink at least eight 8-ounce cups of water
☐ take a multivitamin
☐ eat only lean meats, fish, seafood, nuts, fruits and vegetables
☐ drink 1 serving of a protein shake before breakfast and dinner
☐ enjoy sugars, juice, sweets and soda in moderation
☐ avoid all artificially colored and processed foods

Sheg Aranmolate, MD

day fifty - seven:
our reputation

> A good reputation is more valuable than money.
> <u>Publilius Syrus</u>

One day, my friend called and described how he just bought a brand new car. I immediately asked him to tell me more about his car--the brand, the model and the specifications. My friend proudly answered my questions and told me all the details of his new ride. Upon hearing his answer, I quickly realized why my friend was so excited and proud of his luxurious import. All of us are familiar with brand name products and logos because we are surrounded by them, and because many of the products we use daily are branded with some unique logo. From experience and from watching advertisements we have learned to attach value, quality and even price to items based on their logos. For instance, many of us can see the logo of a car company and estimate the value, price and reputation of that company's cars. In a similar way, our mannerisms and behaviors are very much like logos, and just as we use logos to rapidly assess the quality of a product, other people use our manners and behaviors to judge our character. If you ever had a bad experience with a company, it is likely that this experience will cause you to dislike the company, their products and perhaps even their logos. As a result, every time you see that company's logo, you might be reminded of your bad experience. In the same respect, some of us have damaged our character, or at least the image people have of it, by acting inappropriately or by having obnoxious manners. Please always remember that your reputation belongs to you and it's your responsibility to preserve it. Uphold your reputation like it's your most precious belonging as it's extremely difficult to repair a tarnished image.

workout: chest

☐ incline bench press   [10 reps x 5 times]

weights (lbs):					

☐ decline bench press   [10 reps x 5 times]

weights (lbs):					

☐ flat bench press   [10 reps x 5 times]

weights (lbs):					

☐ pec deck   [10 reps x 5 times]

weights (lbs):					

☐ hammer press   [10 reps x 5 times]

weights (lbs):					

☐ dips   [20 reps x 5 times]

weights (lbs):					

cardio: treadmill

☐ paced walk/jog   [30 minutes]

calories:	

nutrition:

☐ drink at least eight 8-ounce cups of water
☐ take a multivitamin
☐ eat only lean meats, fish, seafood, nuts, fruits and vegetables
☐ drink 1 serving of a protein shake before breakfast and dinner
☐ avoid starches, grains, sugars, juice, sweets and soda
☐ avoid all artificially colored and processed foods

day fifty - eight:
diversification

> If we cannot end now our differences, at least we can help
> make the world safe for diversity.
> John F. Kennedy

Suppose a total stranger asked you why you cherished and enjoyed life, will you be able to a give genuine answer to this question? Honestly, I personally will have a tough time answering such a question because there are too many aspects of life that I cherish. Nevertheless, if I was forced to give an answer, I will say that I cherish and enjoy life because of the beautiful diversity in the world. It is quite obvious that many of us go to the zoo to see exotic animals that we normally don't encounter in our everyday lives. Now, suppose you and your family went to the zoo and after paying the entrance fee, discovered that the entire zoo was populated with only cows. I am quite sure that you will be disappointed and might even demand a refund. It is surprising, then, that many of us are intolerant of human diversity and differences in other people. Indeed, many of us prefer to live around others with similar beliefs, interests and lifestyles. We also often tend to believe that our lifestyles are the best and should be the standard for others. We must remember, however, that if everyone in our society was the same (dressed, looked, spoke and acted the same), then our society will be less interesting and beautiful than it is now. Diversity makes our world an interestingly beautiful place! Please don't be a closed minded individual with rigid convictions--embrace the diversity of persons around you, including their ideas, appearance, culture, musical interests, etc. You will be surprised that such a change will allow you to cherish your time on this beautiful planet that we all consider home.

tasks:

workout: back/traps

☐ deadlift   [10 reps x 5 times]

weights (lbs):					

☐ pulldowns   [10 reps x 5 times]

weights (lbs):					

☐ bent over row   [10 reps x 5 times]

weights (lbs):					

☐ cable row   [10 reps x 5 times]

weights (lbs):					

☐ pull ups   [10 reps x 5 times]

weights (lbs):					

☐ shrugs   [10 reps x 5 times]

weights (lbs):					

cardio: stairmaster

☐ paced walk   [30 minutes]

calories:	

nutrition:

☐ drink at least eight 8-ounce cups of water
☐ take a multivitamin
☐ eat only lean meats, fish, seafood, nuts, fruits and vegetables
☐ drink 1 serving of a protein shake before breakfast and dinner
☐ avoid starches, grains, sugars, juice, sweets and soda
☐ avoid all artificially colored and processed foods

Sheg Aranmolate, MD

day fifty - nine:
emotional projections

> You must learn from the mistakes of others. You can't
> possibly live long enough to make them all yourself.
> <u>Sam Levenson</u>

Late one night, while I was studying for an important chemistry exam, a friend of mine called me and was sobbing because she had just broken up with her boyfriend. She desperately needed my help, so, forgetting my exam, I focused my attention on her and talked to her. As we began talking, I was surprised to hear her anger and resentment toward her boyfriend because there was a time when they were literally inseparable from one another. After talking to her for about two hours, she relaxed and felt better about her situation. Humans are very unique and interesting creatures, and it is amazing how fast our feelings and attitude towards a person can change from love to dislike or hatred in a matter of seconds. When we really like a person, we become excited to be around him or her and everything always seems perfect. For instance, when that person tells a story, we are attentive and quick to laugh at the person's jokes, even when the jokes aren't funny. However, when we dislike a person, everything he or she does puts us on edge. Even simple things like the way the person talks, walks or even smiles can annoy us. The reason for this drastic change is that our emotions largely depend on the actions of other people, and in return we project our emotions on others. Thus, our anger towards people who hurt us reveals itself through our actions and the way we perceive them. Many of us could be less angry with ourselves and with others if we reflected on how we are letting our emotions affect our perception of the world. Nevertheless, avoid getting involved in relationships with people who act badly--they will eventually hurt you.

tasks:

workout: legs

☐ squats   [10 reps x 5 times]

weights (lbs):				

☐ squat to bench   [10 reps x 5 times]

weights (lbs):				

☐ quad extensions   [15 reps x 5 times]

weights (lbs):				

☐ leg curls   [15 reps x 5 times]

weights (lbs):				

☐ leg press calf raises   [20 reps x 5 times]

weights (lbs):				

☐ seated calf raises   [20 reps x 5 times]

weights (lbs):				

cardio: elliptical

☐ paced walk   [30 minutes]

calories:	

nutrition:

☐ drink at least eight 8-ounce cups of water
☐ take a multivitamin
☐ eat only lean meats, fish, seafood, nuts, fruits and vegetables
☐ drink 1 serving of a protein shake before breakfast and dinner
☐ avoid starches, grains, sugars, juice, sweets and soda
☐ avoid all artificially colored and processed foods

day sixty:
cute skunks

> I was always looking outside myself for strength and confidence, but it comes from within. It is there all the time.
> <u>Anna Freud</u>

Skunks are famous for their ability to spray a chemical so potent that it makes large predators run away in disgust. Skunks typically only release this potent scent at times when they are scared or feel threatened by potentially dangerous animals. Besides their capability to produce an intense smell, skunks are actually cute animals. Take a look at several pictures of skunks in the library or online, and you may be surprised to realize that their small heads, petite bodies, and fluffy black and white fur make them really adorable. On a similar note, many people are similar to these adorable skunks. Such people are usually, at first meeting, attractive, nice and cordial. However, as soon as people try to get close to them, they become anxious, show their nasty side, and push others away with their distant behaviors. This erratic behavior is usually due to some painful experiences in life that have made such people inherently distrusting of others. Ironically, many of these people don't always realize that they are actually pushing others away and wonder why they can't be in or form stable relationships. Please don't be like a cute skunk that lures people with looks, only to treat them poorly and spray them with harsh manners. Learn to better understand yourself and other people before making any assumptions so that you don't chase away great people from your life.

tasks:

workout: deltoids

☐ military press behind the neck   [10 reps x 5 times]

weights (lbs):					

☐ military press   [10 reps x 5 times]

weights (lbs):					

☐ dumbbell shoulder press   [10 reps x 5 times]

weights (lbs):					

☐ machine shoulder press   [10 reps x 5 times]

weights (lbs):					

☐ reverse pec deck   [10 reps x 5 times]

weights (lbs):					

☐ dumbbell front raises   [20 reps x 5 times]

weights (lbs):					

cardio: treadmill

☐ paced walk/jog   [30 minutes]

calories:	

nutrition:

☐ drink at least eight 8-ounce cups of water
☐ take a multivitamin
☐ eat only lean meats, fish, seafood, nuts, fruits and vegetables
☐ drink 1 serving of a protein shake before breakfast and dinner
☐ avoid starches, grains, sugars, juice, sweets and soda
☐ avoid all artificially colored and processed foods

Sheg Aranmolate, MD

day sixty - one:
the connoisseur

> The wisest mind has something yet to learn.
> George Santayana

You may have once heard that 'to walk, one must first learn to crawl." This old adage, despite its simplicity, embodies a powerful message, which is that to become proficient in any skill, even one as complex as performing brain surgery, a person must begin as a novice and work up to the proficiency level of an expert. Have you ever thought about how it took several years for us to learn to walk correctly and write without making a mess? Isn't it ironic, then, that many of us are impatient when it comes to learning new ideas and achieving success. The reason many of us fail in trying to start or do new things is that we have already given up on ourselves, even before we started. It is a well-known fact that achieving any form of great or true success isn't an easy task. Nevertheless, enduring through tough times is necessary for us to achieve our goals. What will happen if all babies around the world suddenly stopped trying to walk? Such an event will be a cause for alarm and will be catastrophic to the human race. Fortunately, babies don't give up, and they continually push themselves to get on their own feet--they fall several times but keep pushing until they become successful. Please don't be misguided by get-rich schemes or fad-diets. Success, like any acquired skill, requires tons of sacrifice, dedication and grit. In times of disappointment, always remember that you didn't learn to walk overnight, so don't always expect to manifest all your desires overnight, either.

---

workout: arms/forearms

☐ pushdowns   [10 reps x 5 times]

weights (lbs):					

☐ wide grip curls   [10 reps x 5 times]

weights (lbs):					

☐ cable kickback   [10 reps x 5 times]

weights (lbs):					

☐ seated triceps press   [10 reps x 5 times]

weights (lbs):					

☐ hammer curls   [10 reps x 5 times]

weights (lbs):					

☐ concentration curls   [20 reps x 5 times]

weights (lbs):					

cardio: stairmaster

☐ paced walk   [30 minutes]

calories:	

nutrition:

☐ drink at least eight 8-ounce cups of water
☐ take a multivitamin
☐ eat only lean meats, fish, seafood, nuts, fruits and vegetables
☐ drink 1 serving of a protein shake before breakfast and dinner
☐ avoid starches, grains, sugars, juice, sweets and soda
☐ avoid all artificially colored and processed foods

day sixty - two:
a statistic

There are three kinds of lies: lies, damned lies, and statistics.
Benjamin Disraeli

Companies make billions of dollars in profit yearly on various fitness and weight-loss programs, while the United States government spends billions on weight-related issues. Despite all the profits made and all the money spent, the United States Centers for Disease Control and Prevention estimates that more than half of Americans are overweight, of which more than half that fraction are obese. No one can deny the fact that there are several health problems associated with being overweight such as diabetes, chronic fatigue, brittle bones, shortness of breath and many other issues. It is disheartening that many people on a daily basis are subjected to these debilitating conditions. Of course, there are those whose weight issues are due to their genetic makeup, but most overweight people are in such a state simply due to bad eating habits. It is normal for humans to want to overeat when we have access to a plethora of cheap food, but the effect will often be weight gain. Be honest, have you ever seen an overweight person in those documentaries about famine in other countries? These people are usually extremely thin and bony. However, if these famished individuals were given unlimited access to fatty foods, then many of them will overeat and consequently become overweight too. The function of food is to provide us with the correct nutrients required to function properly, but presently many of us have become habitual eaters who eat to mask true emotions, for enjoyment, or for the sake of eating. If you do this, then you can't keep blaming food for your weight problem. We all have free will and can avoid overeating. Please don't let yourself become a statistic for weight gain. Exercise free will and start living a healthy lifestyle.

---

workout: abs/core

☐ weighted sit ups   [20 reps x 5 times]

weights (lbs):					

☐ weighted cable crunch   [10 reps x 5 times]

weights (lbs):					

☐ leg raises   [20 reps x 5 times]

weights (lbs):					

☐ air bike   [60 reps x 5 times]

weights (lbs):					

☐ side bends   [40 reps x 5 times]

weights (lbs):					

☐ hanging leg raises   [20 reps x 5 times]

weights (lbs):					

cardio: elliptical

☐ paced walk   [30 minutes]

calories:	

nutrition:

☐ drink at least eight 8-ounce cups of water
☐ take a multivitamin
☐ eat only lean meats, fish, seafood, nuts, fruits and vegetables
☐ drink 1 serving of a protein shake before breakfast and dinner
☐ avoid starches, grains, sugars, juice, sweets and soda
☐ avoid all artificially colored and processed foods

day sixty - three:
true fairy tales

> Rarely do great beauty and great virtue dwell together.
> Francesco Petrarch

*C*inderella, *Sleeping Beauty*, and several other fairy tales are inspirational because they teach children and adults alike the triumphant power of good over evil. The story and of Cinderella has a strong correlation to the lives of many of us today. According to the tale, Cinderella was of a noble bloodline, but with the death of her father her family status was reduced. As a result, Cinderella was forced to become a maid and slave for her evil stepmother. Despite adversity, she remained kindhearted and optimistic that her situation would someday improve for the better. After various trials and tribulations, Cinderella came out victorious and lived happily ever after with her Prince Charming. Many of us, like Cinderella, are meant to be living successful lives, but due to unfortunate circumstances we have been unable to improve our situations. We try really hard to climb up the ladder of life, but it always seems like an evil stepmother is thwarting our plans. Then, in an unexpected fashion and like the appearance of the fairy godmother, we encounter a promising opportunity that changes our lives for the better. However, just like Cinderella forgot about the time limit of the fairy godmother's spell, many of us get so carried away by all the glamour of our new lives that we forget our true values, only to be relegated to our previously tough lives. Unlike many of us who might immediately lose hope upon relegation, Cinderella didn't lose faith and in no time was back in the palace. In fact, she didn't even have to look for success because success (in form of the Prince) came looking for her. Please don't lose hope if your life is looking bleak. Your redemption might just be around the corner, looking frantically for you like the Prince searching for the lady with the glass slipper.

---

tasks:

workout: none
☐ rest

cardio: none
☐ rest

nutrition:
☐ drink at least eight 8-ounce cups of water
☐ take a multivitamin
☐ eat only lean meats, fish, seafood, nuts, fruits and vegetables
☐ drink 1 serving of a protein shake before breakfast and dinner
☐ enjoy sugars, juice, sweets and soda in moderation
☐ avoid all artificially colored and processed foods

Sheg Aranmolate, MD

day sixty - four:
different viewpoints

> We can complain because rose bushes have thorns, or
> rejoice because thorn bushes have roses.
> <u>Abraham Lincoln</u>

Whenever I watch a movie, I sometimes enjoy watching the movie blurbs, the "behind-the-scenes" footage, and the director's commentary. These clips take away the larger-than-life feel of most movies and often reveal the true personalities of the performers. Most directors mention how they have to re-shoot certain scenes several times, not because of bad lighting or poor acting from the performers, but rather to get different angles of the same scene, which gives audiences a dynamic view of the acting. In the same accord, we should apply the rationale of directors to re-shoot scenes to our own lives. For example, many of us think that we are living uneventful lives. This is not because we are boring but because we tend to view our lives with a narrow focus rather than with a wide angle lens. As a result, we miss many of the important details that make life worthwhile, like how our advice has helped, our younger siblings or how your idea in class or work gave someone else a different perspective on life. We also tend to become impatient and upset when we feel that we are stalled in life or that we are repeating certain aspects of our lives again (e.g. summer school, a difficult class or the same job). However, similar to a great movie director repeating certain scenes for quality reasons, being stalled or having to repeat certain aspects of our lives again can be a golden opportunity for us to get a better view of our lives and what goals we truly want to pursue. Please treat your life as a vigilant director will treat his or her movie--shoot from many different angles.

---

tasks:

workout: chest

☐ incline bench press   [10 reps x 5 times]

weights (lbs):					

☐ decline bench press   [10 reps x 5 times]

weights (lbs):					

☐ flat bench press   [10 reps x 5 times]

weights (lbs):					

☐ pec deck   [10 reps x 5 times]

weights (lbs):					

☐ hammer press   [10 reps x 5 times]

weights (lbs):					

☐ dips   [20 reps x 5 times]

weights (lbs):					

cardio: treadmill

☐ paced walk/jog   [30 minutes]

calories:	

nutrition:

☐ drink at least eight 8-ounce cups of water
☐ take a multivitamin
☐ eat only lean meats, fish, seafood, nuts, fruits and vegetables
☐ drink 1 serving of a protein shake before breakfast and dinner
☐ avoid starches, grains, sugars, juice, sweets and soda
☐ avoid all artificially colored and processed foods

Sheg Aranmolate, MD

day sixty - five:
a little donation

The strongest principle of growth lies in human choice.
George Eliot

One day Mark, one of my closest friends in America, called from Rwanda, where he had been working for several months with doctors in a hospital. I was excited to hear from my friend and wanted to know about his experiences in Africa. Because of the tragic acts of genocide that occurred there in 1994, I expected to hear horrifying stories about this country. However, to my surprise most of his stories were pretty exciting and interesting. He told me about hikes he took in the rainforest, his safari in Kenya, and his encounters with lions and other exotic animals. He also mentioned how, in recent weeks, he had lost a couple pounds. This was surprising to hear because he was already a pretty slim person. He told me that when he arrived at the village and saw many hungry children, he had decided to give one of his meals each day to a hungry family or a child. Mark said that it was exhilarating to make such a simple sacrifice for so great an effect. Mark's description of his days in Rwanda was very touching and it also made me thinking about the attitude many of us have about fitness and weight-loss. In developed countries, citizens have access to large amounts of food and some go on strict and often excessively caloric restricting diets to temporarily lose a few extra pounds. I came to the conclusion that if everyone in America and other developed countries who are on a diet acted like my friend and gave a meal a day to less fortunate individuals or the money equivalent to meal to a non-profit organization, then both parties (the givers and the receivers) could benefit greatly--the giver with weight loss and the receiver with weight gain.

workout: back/traps

- ☐ deadlift   [10 reps x 5 times]

weights (lbs):					

- ☐ pulldowns   [10 reps x 5 times]

weights (lbs):					

- ☐ bent over row   [10 reps x 5 times]

weights (lbs):					

- ☐ cable row   [10 reps x 5 times]

weights (lbs):					

- ☐ pull ups   [10 reps x 5 times]

weights (lbs):					

- ☐ shrugs   [10 reps x 5 times]

weights (lbs):					

cardio: stairmaster

- ☐ paced walk   [30 minutes]

calories:	

nutrition:

- ☐ drink at least eight 8-ounce cups of water
- ☐ take a multivitamin
- ☐ eat only lean meats, fish, seafood, nuts, fruits and vegetables
- ☐ drink 1 serving of a protein shake before breakfast and dinner
- ☐ avoid starches, grains, sugars, juice, sweets and soda
- ☐ avoid all artificially colored and processed foods

day sixty - six:
opinionated folks

> Everyone rises to their level of incompetence.
> Laurence J. Peter

Nowadays, we can't watch television without seeing a car commercial featuring the latest gadgets and gizmos of newer models. It is undeniable that the low-angle shots of the cars along with the electrifying background music in these commercials usually make the average viewer crave newer models. A vintage car collector, however, might not be intrigued by these commercials. In fact, such a person might consider these commercials as tacky and tasteless. The truth is that different people have different tastes, views and opinions for the same thing. Thus, what you might consider to be appealing might be repulsive to someone else, and vice-versa. Interestingly, it seems like many of us have become oblivious to our differences in taste so that we try to force our opinions on others and will sometimes become upset when others don't agree with them. Many people, especially the young adults, seem frustrated with their lives, mainly because their family members and friends want them to live according to certain standards. Indeed it can be maddening when everyone around appears to be imposing their ideas and standards upon you while disregarding yours. It is important to realize, however, that no one but you can truly know how it feels like to be you and how you are affected by certain opinions. Therefore, it's important that you always have the final say in matters that affect your life. Please don't become someone else's puppet. Take control of your own strings and realize that you are entitled to your own unique taste as long as it doesn't cause harm to others.

tasks:

workout: legs

☐ squats   [10 reps x 5 times]

weights (lbs):				

☐ squat to bench   [10 reps x 5 times]

weights (lbs):				

☐ quad extensions   [15 reps x 5 times]

weights (lbs):				

☐ leg curls   [15 reps x 5 times]

weights (lbs):				

☐ leg press calf raises   [20 reps x 5 times]

weights (lbs):				

☐ seated calf raises   [20 reps x 5 times]

weights (lbs):				

cardio: elliptical

☐ paced walk   [30 minutes]

calories:	

nutrition:

☐ drink at least eight 8-ounce cups of water
☐ take a multivitamin
☐ eat only lean meats, fish, seafood, nuts, fruits and vegetables
☐ drink 1 serving of a protein shake before breakfast and dinner
☐ avoid starches, grains, sugars, juice, sweets and soda
☐ avoid all artificially colored and processed foods

                                           Sheg Aranmolate, MD

day sixty - seven:
unfamiliar territory

> Change your thoughts and you change your world.
> Norman Vincent Peale

When I first learned that I was going to the United States for college, I was excited about the prospect of being independent and free from my parent's control. However, when I first arrived and saw the large college campus, I became nervous and a little homesick. I realized that I was far away from home and in unfamiliar territory. Nevertheless, I knew that there was no turning back and I had to adjust to my new environment. The simple truth about many of us is that we get excited about the idea of changing certain aspects of our lives such as our jobs or location, but become fearful and apprehensive when these changes begin to occur. Change is inevitable in life, and although necessary, it can be difficult and painful at first. For example, every child at some point has to undergo the painful process of losing their baby teeth for stronger permanent teeth. Along the same lines, recent college graduates have to adjust to the work world and young parents have to deal with the new demands and challenges of parenthood. It is important to note, however, that by being positive about the entire experience and with a bit of determination, these life changes can make us stronger and better individuals. Just take a moment to think about it! Humans are adaptable and resourceful by nature, and in time, we can acclimatize to almost any environment. If you are going through changes in your life that seem unbearable, realize that things will eventually get better. You're a member of the resilient human race, which in efforts to explore and adapt to new environments has moved mountains, redirected rivers, built submarines and designed spaceships, simply by changing and applying their thoughts.

tasks:

workout: deltoids

☐ military press behind the neck　　　[10 reps x 5 times]

weights (lbs):					

☐ military press　　　　　　　　　[10 reps x 5 times]

weights (lbs):					

☐ dumbbell shoulder press　　　　[10 reps x 5 times]

weights (lbs):					

☐ machine shoulder press　　　　[10 reps x 5 times]

weights (lbs):					

☐ reverse pec deck　　　　　　　[10 reps x 5 times]

weights (lbs):					

☐ dumbbell front raises　　　　　[20 reps x 5 times]

weights (lbs):					

cardio: treadmill

☐ paced walk/jog　　　　　　　　[30 minutes]

calories:	

nutrition:

☐ drink at least eight 8-ounce cups of water
☐ take a multivitamin
☐ eat only lean meats, fish, seafood, nuts, fruits and vegetables
☐ drink 1 serving of a protein shake before breakfast and dinner
☐ avoid starches, grains, sugars, juice, sweets and soda
☐ avoid all artificially colored and processed foods

day sixty - eight:
trepidation

> Mistakes are the portals of discovery.
> James Joyce

As a youngster, I was so fond of martial arts that I often acted out scenes from the many martial arts movies I saw. Over the years, I concluded that the majority of these movies are about a defeated underdog who--after undergoing rigorous training--becomes victorious in the end. These movies, besides their intense action scenes and sometimes humorous dialogue, taught valuable lessons about the importance of perseverance and the crippling effects our fears. For example, one movie showed how an inexperienced fighter could meditate and train hard enough to beat an expert killer who had enslaved the fighter's village and who had once almost beaten the fighter to death. Many of us face times of great trial and tribulation, such as when we battle deadly addictions, lose our jobs, become bankrupt, fall gravely ill or lose a loved one. These moments can be frightening and can test our willpower. However, the difference between getting through these times and giving up can often be our ability to persevere, which involves controlling our fears. Fear truly has a crippling effect on us! It makes us hesitate and we become vulnerable to making more mistakes. Don't allow your fears to prevent you from getting the upper hand in life. Next time you face a difficult situation that seems to test your might, relax, think logically and control your inner fears. In the end, you might be surprised that it is a lot easier to sail through tough times than you initially thought.

tasks:

workout: arms/forearms

☐ pushdowns   [10 reps x 5 times]

weights (lbs):					

☐ wide grip curls   [10 reps x 5 times]

weights (lbs):					

☐ single arm cable kickbacks   [10 reps x 5 times]

weights (lbs):					

☐ seated triceps press   [10 reps x 5 times]

weights (lbs):					

☐ hammer curls   [10 reps x 5 times]

weights (lbs):					

☐ concentration curls   [20 reps x 5 times]

weights (lbs):					

cardio: stairmaster

☐ paced walk   [30 minutes]

calories:	

nutrition:

☐ drink at least eight 8-ounce cups of water
☐ take a multivitamin
☐ eat only lean meats, fish, seafood, nuts, fruits and vegetables
☐ drink 1 serving of a protein shake before breakfast and dinner
☐ avoid starches, grains, sugars, juice, sweets and soda
☐ avoid all artificially colored and processed foods

day sixty - nine:
crappy roommate

Be modest! It is the kind of pride least likely to offend.
Jules Renard

In graduate school, I instructed an introductory biology lab for undergraduates. I noticed that one of the students was often upset, so at the end of one class I asked her how things were going. It turned out that she was upset with her roommate who was particularly nasty and arrogant towards her. I understood why she could be downhearted as it can be miserable living with an inhospitable person. In an attempt to offer advice, I told her that rather than choosing to become so upset in dealing with her roommate, she should act nicely instead. About a week later, this student thanked me for the advice and said that she already felt better about her situation. She added that her acts of kindness towards her roommate have resulted in fewer confrontations. The truth is that many of us sometimes fail to realize that we often subconsciously impose our state of mind on others around us. For instance, when people are happy they usually want to spread this happiness to others. On the flip side, when people are sad or upset they intentionally or unintentionally want to bring others down as well. If we are around someone in the latter case, we should remind ourselves that no one should be able to ruin our day. The world is filled with so many daunting issues and we could use our attention for positive things such as feeding starving children, assisting the elderly, and helping the less-fortunate. We can't always control the way other people feel inside, but we can control how we feel and deal with those people. Try to treat someone who is treating you poorly with kindness. If all else fails, walk away. Please don't let someone else make you act against your will. Always try to enjoy life and be a dispenser of joy rather than hatred.

workout: abs/core

☐ weighted sit ups   [20 reps x 5 times]

weights (lbs):					

☐ weighted cable crunch   [10 reps x 5 times]

weights (lbs):					

☐ leg raises   [20 reps x 5 times]

weights (lbs):					

☐ air bike   [60 reps x 5 times]

weights (lbs):					

☐ side bends   [40 reps x 5 times]

weights (lbs):					

☐ hanging leg raises   [20 reps x 5 times]

weights (lbs):					

cardio: elliptical

☐ paced walk   [30 minutes]

calories:	

nutrition:

☐ drink at least eight 8-ounce cups of water
☐ take a multivitamin
☐ eat only lean meats, fish, seafood, nuts, fruits and vegetables
☐ drink 1 serving of a protein shake before breakfast and dinner
☐ avoid starches, grains, sugars, juice, sweets and soda
☐ avoid all artificially colored and processed foods

day seventy:
true junkies

Fight for your opinions, but do not believe that they contain the
whole truth, or the only truth.
Charles A. Dana

Many of us have become so addicted to coffee that we literally can't start our days without some. Headaches, fatigue, irritability and restlessness are just a few of the signs of caffeine withdrawal from habitual coffee use. When we think about addicts, we usually think about drug addicts--rarely those addicted to coffee. An addiction is basically a condition in which someone compulsively occupies his or her time with a substance or some activity. Thus, some addicts include sport fanatics, workaholics, and even party animals. An interesting point is that many of us fall into one of the above categories, and it is ironic that we can be quick to judge other addicts and act like we're flawless. From a philosophical point of view, there is little difference between, say, a coffee addict and a cocaine addict because both individuals are dependent on a substance for a stimulus. To better understand drug addicts, we should keep in mind that if some evil-doer forcibly administered an addictive drug like cocaine over time to a random set of people, then many of those subjects would likely develop an addiction to the substance. Given this, we should try to be more tolerant and not judge people who have become addicted to drugs; although we should tell addicts that they have made a grave mistake while helping them to recover. Realize that we all have inherent flaws and weaknesses and we're all prone to making mistakes and developing addictions, just like drug addicts made a grave mistake. It's better to help addicts off their addiction than to waste precious time judging and criticizing. Please if you know someone is addicted to a toxic substance or activity, help them.

tasks:

workout: none
- ☐ rest

cardio: none
- ☐ rest

nutrition:
- ☐ drink at least eight 8-ounce cups of water
- ☐ take a multivitamin
- ☐ eat only lean meats, fish, seafood, nuts, fruits and vegetables
- ☐ drink 1 serving of a protein shake before breakfast and dinner
- ☐ enjoy sugars, juice, sweets and soda in moderation
- ☐ avoid all artificially colored and processed foods

Sheg Aranmolate, MD

day seventy - one:
set the rules

> Laughter gives us distance. It allows us to step back from an
> event, deal with it and then move on.
> <u>Bob Newhart</u>

There's no doubt that you will be out of place if you wore swim trunks to graduation or a tuxedo on a camping trip. Society imposes rules, both explicit and unspoken, with regards to what clothing should be worn for a given occasion. In many situations there can be some flexibility to what we can wear. For instance, we can wear almost anything from a dress shirt to jeans, at a beach party. Nevertheless, one of the reasons we set fashion standards is to prevent our lives from getting mundane and to ensure that we feel special when we dress elaborately. If everyone wore the same clothes all the time, no matter the event, sooner or later our lives will become dull. Unlike with types of clothing in certain situations, we should never treat people with different levels of dignity. It is illogical that many of us have silly rules regarding the way we interact with people. For example, I had a friend who used to be nice to everyone back in his college days. However, after graduating and getting a job, he became cold and distant towards people. This was probably due to his false perception that older, working-class persons are supposed to be serious and unfriendly. It is undeniable that we undergo several behavioral changes as we age and mature, but this shouldn't be a reason to become arrogant or mean-spirited. Life is hard enough! Just like humans need food to live, we need laughter and cheer to help us survive our stressful society. Break the cycle of acting differently to different people--laugh and don't worry about others laughing at you because if everyone is laughing no one will be fighting.

workout: chest

☐ incline bench press   [10 reps x 5 times]

weights (lbs):					

☐ decline bench press   [10 reps x 5 times]

weights (lbs):					

☐ flat bench press   [10 reps x 5 times]

weights (lbs):					

☐ pec deck   [10 reps x 5 times]

weights (lbs):					

☐ hammer press   [10 reps x 5 times]

weights (lbs):					

☐ dips   [20 reps x 5 times]

weights (lbs):					

cardio: treadmill

☐ paced walk/jog   [30 minutes]

calories:	

nutrition:

☐ drink at least eight 8-ounce cups of water
☐ take a multivitamin
☐ eat only lean meats, fish, seafood, nuts, fruits and vegetables
☐ drink 1 serving of a protein shake before breakfast and dinner
☐ avoid starches, grains, sugars, juice, sweets and soda
☐ avoid all artificially colored and processed foods

day seventy - two:
precious ideas

This is my answer to the gap between ideas and action - I will write it out.

Hortense Calisher

I was up late one night in college working frantically on a physics assignment due the next day. One of the mathematical problems was particularly challenging and I spent several hours trying to figure it out. Out of the blue, I thought of the solution but I ended up forgetting it after my friend briefly interrupted my train of thought with a trivial conversation. I was back to square-one--once again, my memory had failed me! There is no doubt that humans can be easily distracted and we occasionally forget certain ideas, thoughts and memories. Sometimes this can be a good thing, such as when we forget painful and traumatic memories. However, we also lose many great ideas that could have benefited us and the world. Distractions are rampant in our busy world and thus it is quite easy for us to be forgetful or sidetracked. But this is no good excuse. Whenever you have a great idea in your head, it is best to act like some of the world's greatest thinkers and write them down before you lose them forever. The biggest differences between humans and other animals in the world include our imagination, ability to think objectively and our desire to transform abstract ideas into reality. As a result, our unique ideas are some of our greatest possessions. They have the ability to change the world and the lives of millions, even billions of people. Please don't take them for granted.

workout: back/traps

☐ deadlift   [10 reps x 5 times]

weights (lbs):					

☐ pulldowns   [10 reps x 5 times]

weights (lbs):					

☐ bent over row   [10 reps x 5 times]

weights (lbs):					

☐ cable row   [10 reps x 5 times]

weights (lbs):					

☐ pull ups   [10 reps x 5 times]

weights (lbs):					

☐ shrugs   [10 reps x 5 times]

weights (lbs):					

cardio: stairmaster

☐ paced walk   [30 minutes]

calories:	

nutrition:

☐ drink at least eight 8-ounce cups of water
☐ take a multivitamin
☐ eat only lean meats, fish, seafood, nuts, fruits and vegetables
☐ drink 1 serving of a protein shake before breakfast and dinner
☐ avoid starches, grains, sugars, juice, sweets and soda
☐ avoid all artificially colored and processed foods

day seventy - three:
resist the crowd

> No one gossips about other people's secret virtues.
> Bertrand Russell

Fraternities and sororities are an integral part of life on most college campuses, and a majority of these organizations were established to install a sense of pride, leadership and excellence in their members. However, nowadays some of these organizations have replaced old values with excessive drinking, hazing and partying. Although I was never a member of any fraternity while in college, I had the opportunity to learn about fraternities and sororities from a number of friends and acquaintances who were pledged members. I learned that several of these people joined not because they truly believed in the values of the organization, but rather out of peer pressure and because they wanted to be recognized as members of a particular group. It's particularly heartbreaking to realize that many of us are so terrified of the idea of being by ourselves that we're willing to sacrifice our beliefs and convictions for acceptance by people with dissimilar views. Why should anyone abandon him or herself in exchange for acceptance? There are times in life when we sometimes get criticized or mocked by other people because of our unique traits or beliefs. However, being different isn't always a bad thing and it shouldn't be a source of embarrassment. For instance, if all the world's great thinkers such as Tesla, Einstein and Marie-Curie were scared of their erratically different ideas, we would not have the great technologies of today. Please don't be an automaton in the crowd who is incapable of reason. Be yourself, think logically, express your individuality and don't join a group because everyone is joining. Only join if you will be yourself or if you want to make a contribution to help other people. Always allow your true identity and personality to shine.

---

tasks:

workout: back/traps

☐ deadlift   [10 reps x 5 times]

weights (lbs):					

☐ pulldowns   [10 reps x 5 times]

weights (lbs):					

☐ bent over row   [10 reps x 5 times]

weights (lbs):					

☐ cable row   [10 reps x 5 times]

weights (lbs):					

☐ pull ups   [10 reps x 5 times]

weights (lbs):					

☐ shrugs   [10 reps x 5 times]

weights (lbs):					

cardio: stairmaster

☐ paced walk   [30 minutes]

calories:	

nutrition:

☐ drink at least eight 8-ounce cups of water
☐ take a multivitamin
☐ eat only lean meats, fish, seafood, nuts, fruits and vegetables
☐ drink 1 serving of a protein shake before breakfast and dinner
☐ avoid starches, grains, sugars, juice, sweets and soda
☐ avoid all artificially colored and processed foods

day seventy - four:
point of reference

> Civilizations in decline are consistently characterised by a
> tendency towards standardization and uniformity.
> Arnold Toynbee

I consider myself a decent freestyle cook, capable of making tasty concoctions of food that are usually irreproducible. Suppose one day, you decided to make an Asian dish with instructions from a cookbook, and after about an hour of sweating in the kitchen, the dish looked pretty tasty. However, as soon as you took a bite you knew that something was amiss. The dish tasted nothing like a similar one you enjoyed in a Chinese restaurant. You were confident that you had followed the instructions correctly but soon realized that you had measured one of the ingredients in pints rather than in ounces. We all know from experience that certain physical properties can be measured with different units. For example, weight can be measured in "pounds" or "grams," and height can be measured in "feet" or "meters." As expected, mistakes will always result if we use the wrong units to measure something. Similarly, many of us get disappointed in life because we measure the level of our success with the wrong measurements. If you ever feel like you are lagging behind in life, make sure that you are using a correct measure of your success. You could easily be using a wrong measure, such as making comparisons of your life with the lives of doctors, celebrities or other highly successful people. Never compare yourself with people who have already climbed to the top! If you do, then you will likely feel inadequate. In fact, comparing your life with the lives of anyone, regardless of their success, is meaningless because no two people are the same. A great measure of your success will be to set realistic goals for yourself and to see how close you come to accomplishing them.

---

workout: legs

☐ squats   [10 reps x 5 times]

weights (lbs):				

☐ squat to bench   [10 reps x 5 times]

weights (lbs):				

☐ quad extensions   [15 reps x 5 times]

weights (lbs):				

☐ leg curls   [15 reps x 5 times]

weights (lbs):				

☐ leg press calf raises   [20 reps x 5 times]

weights (lbs):				

☐ seated calf raises   [20 reps x 5 times]

weights (lbs):				

cardio: elliptical

☐ paced walk   [30 minutes]

calories:	

nutrition:

☐ drink at least eight 8-ounce cups of water
☐ take a multivitamin
☐ eat only lean meats, fish, seafood, nuts, fruits and vegetables
☐ drink 1 serving of a protein shake before breakfast and dinner
☐ avoid starches, grains, sugars, juice, sweets and soda
☐ avoid all artificially colored and processed foods

day seventy - five:
great responsibilities

> Nearly all men can stand adversity, but if you want to test a
> man's character, give him power.
> Abraham Lincoln

As a kid, I loved reading comic books about superheroes because I was astonished and awestruck by the great powers that these superheroes possessed. Sometimes, I would even imagine myself as a superhero, flying around the world and defeating evil. I became so engulfed by the comic characters that I would get upset whenever the darker sides of the superheroes were revealed to the readers. Back then, I used to think that it was impossible for a lifesaving superhero to have a dark side. However, as I got older I began to understand the poisonous effects of power and how it can corrupt virtuous minds. Great power is like a kitchen knife--both should be used with great care for good ends. In the wrong hands, both can be used for evil. It's unarguable that great power can corrupt the mind. Take a look at all power-drunken world leaders who, although perhaps starting off as good people with good intentions, committed unimaginable atrocities to their own people or others. Just like the superheroes in comic books, every one of us has been bestowed, in one way or the other, with great talents to benefit humanity. It is unfortunate and a great loss to humanity that many of us never develop these talents or reach the true potential of our talents because we either don't discover them or we fear the great responsibilities that come with such talents. Please don't allow your indispensible talents and abilities go to waste—take charge and let your talents positively impact the world. On the other hand, it is important to be aware of the intoxicating effects of great talent and power. Always strive to remain humble and virtuous in all you do, regardless of how powerful or famous you might become.

---

tasks:

workout: deltoids

☐ military press behind the neck   [10 reps x 5 times]

weights (lbs):					

☐ military press   [10 reps x 5 times]

weights (lbs):					

☐ dumbbell shoulder press   [10 reps x 5 times]

weights (lbs):					

☐ machine shoulder press   [10 reps x 5 times]

weights (lbs):					

☐ reverse pec deck   [10 reps x 5 times]

weights (lbs):					

☐ dumbbell front raises   [20 reps x 5 times]

weights (lbs):					

cardio: treadmill

☐ paced walk/jog   [30 minutes]

calories:	

nutrition:

☐ drink at least eight 8-ounce cups of water
☐ take a multivitamin
☐ eat only lean meats, fish, seafood, nuts, fruits and vegetables
☐ drink 1 serving of a protein shake before breakfast and dinner
☐ avoid starches, grains, sugars, juice, sweets and soda
☐ avoid all artificially colored and processed foods

day seventy - six:
braggadocio

> Self-respect is the cornerstone of all virtue.
> John Herschel

Kids are usually very fond of their parents and are quick to brag about them. Once, I saw two young boys in the park argue for several minutes about whose father was bigger and stronger. From their intense facial and body expressions, I clearly could tell that the boys were both proud of their fathers' strength. Although from experience I could somewhat relate with the children, but then another part of myself couldn't fully see the point in their intense arguments. The truth is that many of us still act like these young boys and brag unnecessarily about such things as our jobs, relationships and several worldly possessions. Please don't get me wrong, it is quite normal for us to sometimes talk about new purchases or gifts, but if someone does this excessively, then it becomes pretentious and obnoxious. Whenever I see adults bragging about their jobs and material possessions, I often wonder if their arguments are in any way valid. For instance, can a professional golfer claim to be a better athlete than a professional football player? If you are familiar with both sports, then you know that each activity requires different types of athletic and kinesthetic abilities. Similarly, every one of us has unique abilities that help society and further the progress of humanity. For this reason, our society needs the input and effort of every profession to function optimally. Please don't be disheartened or down that your job or profession doesn't sound as prestigious as, say, an engineer, a scientist or a researcher. If our society only had so-called prestigious professions, then it's very likely that society will crumble. For this reason, take pride in whatever you do, but don't become vain because vanity could lead to your downfall and on a large scale can contribute to society's breakdown.

---

tasks:

workout: arms/forearms

☐ pushdowns   [10 reps x 5 times]

weights (lbs):					

☐ wide grip curls   [10 reps x 5 times]

weights (lbs):					

☐ single arm cable kickbacks   [10 reps x 5 times]

weights (lbs):					

☐ seated triceps press   [10 reps x 5 times]

weights (lbs):					

☐ hammer curls   [10 reps x 5 times]

weights (lbs):					

☐ concentration curls   [20 reps x 5 times]

weights (lbs):					

cardio: stairmaster

☐ paced walk   [30 minutes]

calories:	

nutrition:

☐ drink at least eight 8-ounce cups of water
☐ take a multivitamin
☐ eat only lean meats, fish, seafood, nuts, fruits and vegetables
☐ drink 1 serving of a protein shake before breakfast and dinner
☐ avoid starches, grains, sugars, juice, sweets and soda
☐ avoid all artificially colored and processed foods

Sheg Aranmolate, MD

day seventy – seven:
prejudiced bunch

> The greatest of faults, I should say, is to be conscious of
> none.
> Thomas Carlyle

In one of my undergraduate psychology classes there was a woman who sat in the front and consistently interrupted the professor with questions about such things as the weather and professor's fashion sense. Over time, her behavior began to irritate other students to the point that some students would laugh scornfully whenever she spoke. All of this changed, however, when the woman told the entire class her touching story. She had been involved in a terrible car accident that had damaged her brain and left her with severe memory loss, along with the inability to fully control her thoughts and impulse. As a result, she would blurt out most ideas in her head without a filter. She told the class about the pains of rehabilitation and how she was fighting to be normal again. After her emotional speech several students walked up to her and apologized for their prior rudeness and ignorance of her condition. It is undeniable that many of us criticize other people's actions and behaviors, especially when they seem erratic to us. Just like those students who criticized my classmate, many of us are usually ignorant of the condition that we're so quick to judge and criticize. Who are we to judge a person without truly knowing them? This doesn't mean that malicious behaviors should be excused because we don't understand the mind of the perpetrator, rather it means that we should strive to be more objective rather than subjective in our opinions about others. Every now and then we might be right in our initial perceptions, but at times we are also wrong. Please don't be an ignorant person who is quick to point out other's faults. Be tolerant, considerate and wary of your criticisms.

workout: abs/core

☐ weighted sit ups   [20 reps x 5 times]

weights (lbs):					

☐ weighted cable crunch   [10 reps x 5 times]

weights (lbs):					

☐ leg raises   [20 reps x 5 times]

weights (lbs):					

☐ air bike   [60 reps x 5 times]

weights (lbs):					

☐ side bends   [40 reps x 5 times]

weights (lbs):					

☐ hanging leg raises   [20 reps x 5 times]

weights (lbs):					

cardio: elliptical

☐ paced walk   [30 minutes]

calories:	

nutrition:

☐ drink at least eight 8-ounce cups of water
☐ take a multivitamin
☐ eat only lean meats, fish, seafood, nuts, fruits and vegetables
☐ drink 1 serving of a protein shake before breakfast and dinner
☐ avoid starches, grains, sugars, juice, sweets and soda
☐ avoid all artificially colored and processed foods

day seventy - eight:
visualizing

> Imagination is more important than knowledge.
> Albert Einstein

As a child, remember when it was close to your birthday and you wished that your parents would buy all the toys that you wanted? Of course, most of us had this wish. It was so strong that we would even "unintentionally" express our desires to our parents by, for instance, talking about the toys everyday, drawing pictures of the toys on the wall, and even screaming every time we see the toys on the television. Like the laws of magnetism, it is quite amazing that our parents were compelled (probably out of frustration) to buy at least some of those toys for us. Clearly, as children we could easily visualize our goals and take the necessary steps to achieve them. How come, as we get older and become adults, we forget about or fail to use this ability to be successful? Visualization is a powerful mental tool that only humans possess. It allows us to make a mental image of our desires and develop the appropriate plans and steps needed to realize them. If you doubt the power of visualization, just think about how far we've come along as a species and how much we have accomplished since the Stone Age. If we lacked the ability to visualize, then we will not have all the incredible inventions of today such as cars, houses, airplanes, phones and computers. Even cooking a simple meal in the kitchen like scrambled eggs requires elements of visualization. Most successful people in the world became successful because of their unwavering ability to visualize success and the different ways to obtain it. The truth is that we all have this amazing ability but it is unfortunate that many of us don't use it to our full potential. We all have goal and aspirations. That is why we must tap into our ability to visualize the world we desire. With hard work those thoughts will become reality!

tasks:

workout: none
- ☐ rest

cardio: none
- ☐ rest

nutrition:
- ☐ drink at least eight 8-ounce cups of water
- ☐ take a multivitamin
- ☐ eat only lean meats, fish, seafood, nuts, fruits and vegetables
- ☐ drink 1 serving of a protein shake before breakfast and dinner
- ☐ enjoy sugars, juice, sweets and soda in moderation
- ☐ avoid all artificially colored and processed foods

Sheg Aranmolate, MD

day seventy - nine:
good people

It is pretty hard to tell what does bring happiness; poverty
and wealth have both failed.
Kin Hubbard

One day I was talking to an associate of mine and he told me that he was depressed because he felt the world was filled with much hate and very little inspiration. I disagreed with his extreme view of the world and tried to help him think more positively. I understood that his sadness and feelings of hopelessness were distorting his perception of life and reality. News stories about crime and societal mishaps are reminders that we live in a society which has its share of vindictive people who are out to hurt others. On the other hand and as I told my associate, a quick review of the multitudes of people who work daily for charities and help the needy shows that society is also filled with many kindhearted people who are genuinely have an interest in helping others. Our world is such a beautiful place with so many sources of inspiration. It is unfortunate, however, that many of us sometimes fail to notice them, perhaps because we are in the habit of thinking that sources of inspiration have to be grand in nature. Just take a look at nice people, playing dogs, colorful birds, blue sky, intricate buildings and even sleek cars. What do you think? Are not many sources of inspiration quite common? The fact that humans, from raw materials, designed and built all the existing technologies that we currently enjoy is inspirational in itself. Furthermore, even from a genetic viewpoint, humans are so complex in our inner workings that physicians and scientists alike have yet to fully grasp all the minute details of our bodies. As a result, the indisputable truth is that every human being by right is a living source of inspiration. Find motivation in yourself, use your talents to inspire others, and you will be surprised to find that the more you inspire others, the more inspired you will become.

workout: chest

☐ incline bench press   [10 reps x 5 times]

weights (lbs):					

☐ decline bench press   [10 reps x 5 times]

weights (lbs):					

☐ flat bench press   [10 reps x 5 times]

weights (lbs):					

☐ pec deck   [10 reps x 5 times]

weights (lbs):					

☐ hammer press   [10 reps x 5 times]

weights (lbs):					

☐ dips   [20 reps x 5 times]

weights (lbs):					

cardio: treadmill

☐ paced walk/jog   [30 minutes]

calories:	

nutrition:

☐ drink at least eight 8-ounce cups of water
☐ take a multivitamin
☐ eat only lean meats, fish, seafood, nuts, fruits and vegetables
☐ drink 1 serving of a protein shake before breakfast and dinner
☐ avoid starches, grains, sugars, juice, sweets and soda
☐ avoid all artificially colored and processed foods

day eighty:
the human puzzle

So long as we live among men, let us cherish humanity.
Andre Gide

In college I used to be a resident assistant, and I was in part responsible for the upkeep and maintenance of a floor in the one of the residential halls. At the start of every school year, the resident assistants had to attend an off-campus ropes course to help build an atmosphere of cooperation and teamwork. Activities at the obstacle course included races, rock climbing and a game that involved the formation of a human crossword puzzle. In this puzzle game, every participant was assigned a letter of the alphabet and had to fit in somewhere to complete the answer to a question. The first time I played, I was amazed by how fast we all scrambled around and found our correct positions, although there were several personality clashes. As in this game, we all fit together like a complex jigsaw puzzle in the grand functioning. Every one of us, in a unique way, is required to make a contribution to the lives of others. It's a shame that many of us can be quick to discriminate against others because of an unwarranted sense of entitlement or superiority over others. Just as every piece of a jigsaw puzzle is needed for the complete picture, all of us are important and we each play an essential role that is needed for a functioning society. Can you have one part of a car engine like the pistons or the transmission without the other parts and still have a functioning automobile? No way! From a creative stance, we are all like the words in a great poem, whereby removing a single word throws everything off. As a result, we shouldn't discriminate against others for superficial reasons. Please always remember that in the grand scheme of life you and everyone else are each important in your own way.

tasks:

workout: back/traps

☐ deadlift   [10 reps x 5 times]

weights (lbs):					

☐ pulldowns   [10 reps x 5 times]

weights (lbs):					

☐ bent over row   [10 reps x 5 times]

weights (lbs):					

☐ cable row   [10 reps x 5 times]

weights (lbs):					

☐ pull ups   [10 reps x 5 times]

weights (lbs):					

☐ shrugs   [10 reps x 5 times]

weights (lbs):					

cardio: stairmaster

☐ paced walk   [30 minutes]

calories:	

nutrition:

☐ drink at least eight 8-ounce cups of water
☐ take a multivitamin
☐ eat only lean meats, fish, seafood, nuts, fruits and vegetables
☐ drink 1 serving of a protein shake before breakfast and dinner
☐ avoid starches, grains, sugars, juice, sweets and soda
☐ avoid all artificially colored and processed foods

Sheg Aranmolate, MD

day eighty - one:
mindless zombies

> I have never met a man so ignorant that I couldn't learn
> something from him.
> Galileo Galilei

One time my friends and I watched a horror movie about zombies taking over the world and consequently preying on humans for food. My friends were terrified of the zombies, but I chuckled or laughed loudly when they came onto the screen. I personally find zombie movies quite comical and not scary. This may be because I have seen a number of low budget zombie movies over the years that failed to arouse any form of fear inside of me. Nevertheless, I found it quite interesting how my friends and I reacted differently to the same movie. How could they be frightened by actors and actresses who wore rags, masks and lots of makeup? This just further emphasizes the obvious: that we are all different and can have a wide range of emotions even to the same stimulus. Rarely do we all feel or act the same in a given situation. For instance, some people weep with the loss of a loved one and some people don't. Nevertheless, many of us still act oblivious to this fact and become upset when others don't act or react similarly to ourselves. The truth is that we can't force others to be like ourselves--this is impossible! In fact, if everyone acted and responded similarly, then we will all be like zombies in those movies, incapable of reason and driven by the most basic of impulses. Please don't be like one of those mindless zombies whose sole purpose, if any, is to change everyone to zombies as well. Learn from others' differences and use those differences to better understand your own uniqueness. This simple gesture will likely save you a lot of heartache and disappointment in life.

tasks:

workout: legs

☐ squats   [10 reps x 5 times]

weights (lbs):				

☐ squat to bench   [10 reps x 5 times]

weights (lbs):				

☐ quad extensions   [15 reps x 5 times]

weights (lbs):				

☐ leg curls   [15 reps x 5 times]

weights (lbs):				

☐ leg press calf raises   [20 reps x 5 times]

weights (lbs):				

☐ seated calf raises   [20 reps x 5 times]

weights (lbs):				

cardio: elliptical

☐ paced walk   [30 minutes]

calories:	

nutrition:

☐ drink at least eight 8-ounce cups of water
☐ take a multivitamin
☐ eat only lean meats, fish, seafood, nuts, fruits and vegetables
☐ drink 1 serving of a protein shake before breakfast and dinner
☐ avoid starches, grains, sugars, juice, sweets and soda
☐ avoid all artificially colored and processed foods

                                           Sheg Aranmolate, MD

day eighty - two:
the scornful

> Envy is the ulcer of the soul.
>
> <u>Socrates</u>

Obviously, the world is a diverse collection of people with different traits, personalities, talents and ideas. Therefore, it is not surprising that two people can have opposite views and opinions on the same issue. For example, an optimist will say that the world is at least half-filled with good people who truly care about others, and a pessimist will say that the majority of the world is filled with bad people who are compelled to hurt others. Which of these views is more accurate? The truth of either view seems quite impossible to prove. One thing in the world, however, is much easier to prove, and that is the existence of moral truths. The fact that there are certain acts that we all agree are evil, such as rape and genocide, means that there are moral truths. One person might view a deed as good and someone else might view that deed as evil, but this is not to say that both people are right. It is quite unfortunate that some people have become so engulfed with hatred that they allow it to control their lives and shroud their ability to recognize moral truths. Hatred is like a deep cut on a leg! If cleaned quickly and properly will heal but if left untreated will become infected and detrimental to the entire body. Having hatred for other people, regardless of the cause or reason, results in self-hatred, and this often leads to self destruction. It is important that we never let any kind of hatred control our life and transform us from kindhearted people into persons who act without a conscience. Please practice compassion, be nice to others, and stay clear of hateful people because of the contagious nature of a hateful heart.

tasks:

workout: deltoids

☐ military press behind the neck   [10 reps x 5 times]

weights (lbs):					

☐ military press   [10 reps x 5 times]

weights (lbs):					

☐ dumbbell shoulder press   [10 reps x 5 times]

weights (lbs):					

☐ machine shoulder press   [10 reps x 5 times]

weights (lbs):					

☐ reverse pec deck   [10 reps x 5 times]

weights (lbs):					

☐ dumbbell front raises   [20 reps x 5 times]

weights (lbs):					

cardio: treadmill

☐ paced walk/jog   [30 minutes]

calories:	

nutrition:

☐ drink at least eight 8-ounce cups of water
☐ take a multivitamin
☐ eat only lean meats, fish, seafood, nuts, fruits and vegetables
☐ drink 1 serving of a protein shake before breakfast and dinner
☐ avoid starches, grains, sugars, juice, sweets and soda
☐ avoid all artificially colored and processed foods

Sheg Aranmolate, MD

day eighty - three:
the masterpiece

> Small opportunities are often the beginning of great
> enterprises.
> Demosthenes

My father, besides being a physician, often loved to draw people and animals. As a young chap, I enjoyed watching him draw and listening to him talk about many great artists like Leonardo da Vinci and Pablo Picasso, and how these artists used their imaginations and skills to produce great works of art. My father stressed the fact that anyone can learn to draw well, just like anyone can learn the principles of good writing. I know that, to a large extent, my father was correct in his analysis. The truth is that if every one of us practiced drawing everyday and continually developed our imaginations, the world would be filled with many more great artists. Indeed, practice may not always achieve perfection, but we should strive to become great at what we pursue in life. This usually requires us to put substantial effort into our endeavors and maximize the use our imagination, which, unfortunately, many of us don't realize. The difference between a mediocre artist and a great artist can often be their comparative capacity for imagination. Say two artists of equal physical talent were given the same paints and brushes and told to paint the same scene outside a window. It's unlikely that both artists would paint identical pictures--the quality of the paintings would largely be dependent upon the imagination of the artists. Similarly, many of us are given opportunities to succeed in life, and, like the artists, our chances of coming out on top are often dependent upon our imaginations and persistence. Please don't take life for granted. It is important that you seize every opportunity and use it to produce historic masterpieces in your field, much as the great da Vinci did in his time.

tasks:

workout: arms/forearms

☐ pushdowns   [10 reps x 5 times]

weights (lbs):					

☐ wide grip curls   [10 reps x 5 times]

weights (lbs):					

☐ single arm cable kickbacks   [10 reps x 5 times]

weights (lbs):					

☐ seated triceps press   [10 reps x 5 times]

weights (lbs):					

☐ hammer curls   [10 reps x 5 times]

weights (lbs):					

☐ concentration curls   [20 reps x 5 times]

weights (lbs):					

cardio: stairmaster

☐ paced walk   [30 minutes]

calories:	

nutrition:

☐ drink at least eight 8-ounce cups of water
☐ take a multivitamin
☐ eat only lean meats, fish, seafood, nuts, fruits and vegetables
☐ drink 1 serving of a protein shake before breakfast and dinner
☐ avoid starches, grains, sugars, juice, sweets and soda
☐ avoid all artificially colored and processed foods

Sheg Aranmolate, MD

day eighty - four:
party planners

> Everything you can imagine is real.
> Pablo Picasso

Occassionally I like to have family and friends over to my place for a nice gathering and fellowship. Anyone who has ever hosted a party should know that proper planning is required for a successful event. I have come to realize that there is a big similarity between how we organize parties and how other people in our society strive to help us attain and accomplish our goals. Just as when you take the initiative to apply to college and your state government might offer you grants or scholarships, every time I propose the idea of having a party with my friends they often help make the party a reality by doing such essential things like calling people, setting up party decorations, and buying food and drinks. In an interesting and unique way, many of us seem forgetful about the fact that our ideas and actions have similar power to influence and compel others into helping us accomplish our goals. If we really want to achieve our positive goals and we actively think about them, then our thoughts will eventually help make paths for us to achieve our goals. Think about one thing that you want to accomplish today. What steps are needed for its completion? Does it require only effort on your part or do you need to tap into the strengths of others around you? This simple mental task reveals the power of our thoughts and ability to call on others for assistance. It is quite unfortunate, however, that many of us don't do this and never get to execute or accomplish our desired goals. Please don't keep your goals or aspirations locked up in your head! Our ideas are like perfume scents that, when sprayed, catch people's attention and can influence their actions. Never waste your ideas or goals. Instead, begin to actively ponder and act on them. You will be amazed that people, including strangers, will start working eagerly to help you.

tasks:

workout: abs/core

☐ weighted sit ups   [20 reps x 5 times]

weights (lbs):					

☐ weighted cable crunch   [10 reps x 5 times]

weights (lbs):					

☐ leg raises   [20 reps x 5 times]

weights (lbs):					

☐ air bike   [60 reps x 5 times]

weights (lbs):					

☐ side bends   [40 reps x 5 times]

weights (lbs):					

☐ hanging leg raises   [20 reps x 5 times]

weights (lbs):					

cardio: elliptical

☐ paced walk   [30 minutes]

calories:	

nutrition:

☐ drink at least eight 8-ounce cups of water
☐ take a multivitamin
☐ eat only lean meats, fish, seafood, nuts, fruits and vegetables
☐ drink 1 serving of a protein shake before breakfast and dinner
☐ avoid starches, grains, sugars, juice, sweets and soda
☐ avoid all artificially colored and processed foods

Sheg Aranmolate, MD

day eighty - five:
unlimited desire

> Prediction is very difficult, especially about the future.
> <u>Niels Bohr</u>

When I was younger, I once followed my parents to a buffet lunch at an elegant party. I remember becoming so excited when I saw all the food that I immediately dashed towards the table to literally eat all that I could eat. My excitement and desire, however, was curtailed by my mother, who had decided to ration my portions. As she walked around the table filling my plate, my eyes drifted to a tasty looking shrimp dish, and I begged my mother for a taste. Although she sternly refused my request, I was grateful to her later on because most people at the buffet, including my dad, got terribly sick from eating the shrimp. Humans by nature have a plethora of desires, and it is normal for us to become upset when we don't get the things we want-- I know I fussed at first about the shrimp. Many of us also don't realize that some of our missed opportunities in life have been life savers and have prevented from being entangled in undesirable settings that are not conducive for our optimal growth. For instance, some of us are upset because we have not gotten all our immediate wishes such those weapons, motorcycles or sport cars that we have always wanted, and this has probably saved our health or even lives in some way. On the other hand, because we never get physically or emotionally hurt, many of us never realize how those missed opportunities saved our lives. Let's be quite honest with ourselves! Disappointments in life can be a real bummer, but many of them can also be blessings in disguise. Besides, disappointments can be a subtle sign that we are not yet equipped or fully prepared for the demands and responsibilities associated with the missed opportunity or desire. Next time that you are disappointed or upset about missed opportunities, just keep this in mind: your life might have been a lot worse and you have had some time to be better prepared for the next opportunity.

---

tasks:

workout: none
☐ rest

cardio: none
☐ rest

nutrition:
☐ drink at least eight 8-ounce cups of water
☐ take a multivitamin
☐ eat only lean meats, fish, seafood, nuts, fruits and vegetables
☐ drink 1 serving of a protein shake before breakfast and dinner
☐ enjoy sugars, juice, sweets and soda in moderation
☐ avoid all artificially colored and processed foods

Sheg Aranmolate, MD

day eighty - six:
emotion detectives

> Feel the fear and do it anyway.
> <u>Susan Jeffers</u>

Dogs are great human companions, capable of following detailed instructions and learning complex tasks. When watching cop shows on the television, I always find it fascinating to watch police dogs take down criminals and smell narcotics in the strangest hiding places. From experience, it is quite obvious to many that dogs have a keen sense of smell that is much greater than that of humans, and as a result dogs can recognize a wide range and intensity of odors that we can't. I have even heard that some dogs' sense of smell is so great that they can smell human emotions such as love, compassion, hatred, confidence and even fear. Although we don't rely on our noses, humans are similar to dogs in that we can sense or predict other people's emotions. We can, for the most part, tell when others are sad, happy or nervous. Many of us, however, also seem to forget the fact that the way we perceive ourselves strongly determines the way others perceive us. For example, if you walked into a grocery store and act unkindly towards others then many of them will view and treat you as an unkind person. In a similar manner, if you act and speak confidently towards others then they will likely view and treat you as secure rather than as an insecure person. Also just like in the wild where predators prey on weak animals, people with low self-esteem are often taken advantage of by others who sense their insecurities and who exploit their weaknesses. I'm not implying that we should always be brass and defensive in our daily actions and moods, but rather, we should always strive to bring forth the best of our emotions and confidence. Please don't let others take advantage of you because you're radiating fear. It is important that you change your perception and change your world!

---

tasks:

workout: chest

☐ incline bench press　　　　　　[10 reps x 5 times]

weights (lbs):					

☐ decline bench press　　　　　　[10 reps x 5 times]

weights (lbs):					

☐ flat bench press　　　　　　　[10 reps x 5 times]

weights (lbs):					

☐ pec deck　　　　　　　　　　[10 reps x 5 times]

weights (lbs):					

☐ hammer press　　　　　　　　[10 reps x 5 times]

weights (lbs):					

☐ dips　　　　　　　　　　　　[20 reps x 5 times]

weights (lbs):					

cardio: treadmill

☐ paced walk/jog　　　　　　　[30 minutes]

calories:	

nutrition:

☐ drink at least eight 8-ounce cups of water
☐ take a multivitamin
☐ eat only lean meats, fish, seafood, nuts, fruits and vegetables
☐ drink 1 serving of a protein shake before breakfast and dinner
☐ avoid starches, grains, sugars, juice, sweets and soda
☐ avoid all artificially colored and processed foods

Sheg Aranmolate, MD

day eighty - seven:
impenitent

> The most perfidious way of harming a cause consists of
> defending it deliberately with faulty arguments.
> Friedrich Nietzsche

O nce, I was shopping in the mall for a pair of jeans when a family of five walked into the store. As soon as the parents began shopping, the kids started running around the tables in the store and screaming at the top of their lungs. The kids even knocked down one of the store mannequins, and instead of acknowledging their mess, they continued with their unimpeded ruckus. Their parents were obviously embarrassed and, after picking up the mannequin, scolded their kids. The parents urged the kids to apologize for their actions but they surprisingly refused to say 'sorry" to the store clerk. Not too long afterwards, the family left the store in embarrassment without getting what they had come into the store to buy. It is an undeniable fact that most children are curious, playful, adorable, humorous and boiling over with passionate energy. Unruly kids in public, however, can be quite bothersome and many of us get irritated by these kids, especially when they are unapologetic for their disruptive behaviors. On the other hand, we must all realize that kids learn their behavior from older individuals around them, and that also includes being unapologetic. In the same accord, it is important that we all must be better examples to younger people and be willing to apologize when wrong. In no way should we ever feel that the act of apologizing or admitting our faults makes us look weak or foolish. In fact, doing this makes us more respectable in the eyes of others because the act of apologizing often requires humility and courage. It takes more effort to refuse to apologize or to try and rationalize our bad actions. Please don't be that person who refuses to apologize to others like the boisterous kids in the store because you'll likely end up missing out on great people and prospects in life. Mend your wrong ways!

---

workout: back/traps

☐ deadlift   [10 reps x 5 times]

weights (lbs):					

☐ pulldowns   [10 reps x 5 times]

weights (lbs):					

☐ bent over row   [10 reps x 5 times]

weights (lbs):					

☐ cable row   [10 reps x 5 times]

weights (lbs):					

☐ pull ups   [10 reps x 5 times]

weights (lbs):					

☐ shrugs   [10 reps x 5 times]

weights (lbs):					

cardio: stairmaster

☐ paced walk   [30 minutes]

calories:	

nutrition:

☐ drink at least eight 8-ounce cups of water
☐ take a multivitamin
☐ eat only lean meats, fish, seafood, nuts, fruits and vegetables
☐ drink 1 serving of a protein shake before breakfast and dinner
☐ avoid starches, grains, sugars, juice, sweets and soda
☐ avoid all artificially colored and processed foods

day eighty - eight:
the latent flames

> Hate no one; hate their vices, not themselves.
> J. G. C. Brainard

I will never forget the excitement I felt when I moved from my restrictive dorm room to my very own apartment. A number of the benefits filled my thoughts, like not having to park miles away and not having to deal with noisy college roommates. This move occurred in the start of summer, and after settling in my apartment I learned that it lacked a ceiling fan or air conditioning. After a few scorching nights I soon wished I was back in the comfort of my air-conditioned dorm room. One evening the heat became so unbearable that I called a service technician for assistance. After inspecting my residence, the technician informed me that the intense heat was due to the summer heat in combination with the heat emitted from the natural gas heating unit, which was designed to continuously burn at a low level even during the summers. Upon finding out this news that I would be cooped up in a heat trap all summer, I became very angry at my landlord, who never informed me of the heating problem prior to my signing the lease. Nevertheless, it was a learning experience because, after a while, I learned how to control my anger and to control myself from projecting my frustrations on others. In a unique way, our anger can be like the flames of the heating unit, which lay dim until given more propane. In addition, just as heating units have thermostats that measure the temperature and adjust the intensity of the flames accordingly, we have the ability to control the levels and expression of our anger. Next time you're provoked, take a few minutes before you react to think of the consequences of acting on your anger and let this be a guide. Although it is easier said than done, we should never let any person, object or situation steal our joy and make our anger explode uncontrollably.

---

tasks:

workout: legs

☐ squats [10 reps x 5 times]

weights (lbs):				

☐ squat to bench [10 reps x 5 times]

weights (lbs):				

☐ quad extensions [15 reps x 5 times]

weights (lbs):				

☐ leg curls [15 reps x 5 times]

weights (lbs):				

☐ leg press calf raises [20 reps x 5 times]

weights (lbs):				

☐ seated calf raises [20 reps x 5 times]

weights (lbs):				

cardio: elliptical

☐ paced walk [30 minutes]

calories:	

nutrition:

☐ drink at least eight 8-ounce cups of water
☐ take a multivitamin
☐ eat only lean meats, fish, seafood, nuts, fruits and vegetables
☐ drink 1 serving of a protein shake before breakfast and dinner
☐ avoid starches, grains, sugars, juice, sweets and soda
☐ avoid all artificially colored and processed foods

Sheg Aranmolate, MD

day eighty - nine:
seeking attention

> The joy of a spirit is the measure of its power.
> <u>Ninon de Lenclos</u>

While I was in college, I worked as a valet near Washington, D.C. and I had the opportunity to drive the cars of several senators and business executives. Although, stressful at times with a few humiliating moments, the job was fun because I got to drive several expensive cars and at the same time learn about the unique correlation between flashy cars and flashy people. I noticed that a number of people with expensive cars loved to brag and for the most part appeared to care more about their cars than about the valets driving them. It is valid to say that many of us buy expensive cars both for the luxury features and for the attention that such cars attract. As a result, many of us, when we see an expensive car, often assume that the owner is affluent. However, this isn't always the case because many people who are in serious debt drive expensive cars for the craved attention. Humans love attention by nature and this is shown in the way we dress, talk, and act. Unfortunately, many of us have become so engulfed by our materialistic society that we feel that we can't even be noticed by others until we own the latest clothes, gadgets and gizmos. However, we must realize that we don't need to have all the new stuff to be noticed by others. Whatever happened to sharing a genuine smile, nice gestures, or a hearty laugh with someone? These beautiful and free manners are what really get us noticed. The truth is that you can own the best attire, but if you don't have a good attitude to complement it, then you blend in with the superficial world. A beautiful smile and good gesture are like new jewelry that sparkles in the light but can lose its luster if misused. Be genuine and sparkle with your gleaming smile and great attitude. This will get you all the positive attention that you desire.

---

tasks:

workout: deltoids

☐ military press behind the neck   [10 reps x 5 times]

weights (lbs):					

☐ military press   [10 reps x 5 times]

weights (lbs):					

☐ dumbbell shoulder press   [10 reps x 5 times]

weights (lbs):					

☐ machine shoulder press   [10 reps x 5 times]

weights (lbs):					

☐ reverse pec deck   [10 reps x 5 times]

weights (lbs):					

☐ dumbbell front raises   [20 reps x 5 times]

weights (lbs):					

cardio: treadmill

☐ paced walk/jog   [30 minutes]

calories:	

nutrition:

☐ drink at least eight 8-ounce cups of water
☐ take a multivitamin
☐ eat only lean meats, fish, seafood, nuts, fruits and vegetables
☐ drink 1 serving of a protein shake before breakfast and dinner
☐ avoid starches, grains, sugars, juice, sweets and soda
☐ avoid all artificially colored and processed foods

Sheg Aranmolate, MD

day ninety:
right directions

The best way to predict the future is to invent it.
Alan Kay

Think about this: it was only a few years ago that drivers had to rely on maps on large paper to get directions. Nowadays, we can use online maps to get directions in a matter of seconds. With the emergence of the internet and Global Positioning System (GPS) technology, paper maps have become obsolete. Why should anyone do all the work involved in reading a paper map when with a few strokes on a computer keyboard or smartphone, you can get all the directions you need, even with live traffic updates? Nevertheless, even with all this modern help, many of us at times still get lost or lose time on trips because of wrong turns or inattention. Our journey through life shares many similarities with driving in traffic using online directions. Just as many of us can be overly confident in relying on online directions to get us places, we can become overly confident in our abilities and the direction that our lives are going. In pursuing our goals, we can take wrong turns or get distracted by other people, things or situations and end up losing our way or finding ourselves at unexpected destinations. There are also times when our journey gets detoured due to a number of circumstances beyond our control such as the mistakes of other drivers, unplanned accidents or problems with the road itself. The world is dynamic and filled with many variables, and at times our choices might appear to be out of our hands, but this can lead us to an even better destination than we previously planned. In those unforeseen times, it is important that we keep our cool, remain focused on our destination and make the best out of emergent situations. We must also not be frazzled and get into the habit of periodic self-reflection to make sure that we are where we actually want to be in life. As with following online directions, don't be afraid to stop and ask others for guidance or to trust your own instincts.

tasks:

workout: arms/forearms

☐ pushdowns   [10 reps x 5 times]

weights (lbs):					

☐ wide grip curls   [10 reps x 5 times]

weights (lbs):					

☐ single arm cable kickbacks   [10 reps x 5 times]

weights (lbs):					

☐ seated triceps press   [10 reps x 5 times]

weights (lbs):					

☐ hammer curls   [10 reps x 5 times]

weights (lbs):					

☐ concentration curls   [20 reps x 5 times]

weights (lbs):					

cardio: stairmaster

☐ paced walk   [30 minutes]

calories:	

nutrition:

☐ drink at least eight 8-ounce cups of water
☐ take a multivitamin
☐ eat only lean meats, fish, seafood, nuts, fruits and vegetables
☐ drink 1 serving of a protein shake before breakfast and dinner
☐ avoid starches, grains, sugars, juice, sweets and soda
☐ avoid all artificially colored and processed foods

Sheg Aranmolate, MD

day ninety - one:
similar happiness

> If you want others to be happy, practice compassion. If you want to be happy, practice compassion.
>
> Tenzin Gyatso

When I was young boy, my dog Murphy often accompanied me on my way to school in the morning. When I was near the school entrance he would begin to whine in sadness, and when I would arrive home later he would wag his tail and bark with excitement. Surely, many of us have experienced this with our dogs. It is quite obvious from these gestures that our dogs enjoy our presence, but can we know with certainty that our dogs experience happiness? Whatever excitement Murphy felt was genuine and it made me feel happy about myself, but since dogs cannot speak human languages I will never know about the true emotions, if any, that she truly felt. What I do know is that all humans are capable of experiencing happiness. Some people, due to various circumstances and experiences, say it can be difficult to find reasons in life to be happy or that happiness is a false reality. If an alien from a different planet asked you to explain happiness and to give ten reasons why anyone should be happy, will you be able to give an answer? I personally will not be able to provide a full answer, but I will say that, to become happy, we must identify the proverbial keys to happiness, such as being kind to others, displaying compassionate, selflessness, and humility, and we must at all times pursue and utilize these notions. We are all familiar with the maxim 'practice makes perfect." In the same respect, happiness is like any ability that requires constant practice for proficiency and to reach a state of perfection. Thus, the more you pursue and use the keys of happiness, the greater the odds that you will experience happiness. Pursue those keys today!

workout: abs/core

☐ weighted sit ups   [20 reps x 5 times]

weights (lbs):					

☐ weighted cable crunch   [10 reps x 5 times]

weights (lbs):					

☐ leg raises   [20 reps x 5 times]

weights (lbs):					

☐ air bike   [60 reps x 5 times]

weights (lbs):					

☐ side bends   [40 reps x 5 times]

weights (lbs):					

☐ hanging leg raises   [20 reps x 5 times]

weights (lbs):					

cardio: elliptical

☐ paced walk   [30 minutes]

calories:	

nutrition:

☐ drink at least eight 8-ounce cups of water
☐ take a multivitamin
☐ eat only lean meats, fish, seafood, nuts, fruits and vegetables
☐ drink 1 serving of a protein shake before breakfast and dinner
☐ avoid starches, grains, sugars, juice, sweets and soda
☐ avoid all artificially colored and processed foods

day ninety - two:
vaulted memories

> One must have a good memory to be able to keep the
> promises one makes.
> Friedrich Nietzsche

When we meet people for the first time, we usually shake their hand and say our names. This may seem like a simple gesture, but this gesture involves many complicated mental and physical processes. For instance, when we meet someone we remember his or her face, the circumstances of the meeting, other people who were present, and, if we are lucky, we remember his or her name. The ability to form memories is clearly a large part of life, and it's not an exaggeration to conclude that the human experience is based on our interaction with previously acquired precious memories--both good and bad. Our memories are like files in a file cabinet that are ready for us to retrieve. On a daily basis, there are moments when we can't recall memories or parts of memories. These moments can be frustrating, especially when you know that the memory or part of the memory was a good one and it contained vital information that you needed to accomplish a certain task. Even though this can happen to anyone, it is unfortunate that many of us are quick to get annoyed, angry or frustrated with people who have varying degrees of memory loss. However, just as every one of us is susceptible to catching the same diseases, all of us are susceptible to someday experiencing severe memory loss, either by an accident, prolonged self-abuse or genetic makeup. The truth is that our formed memories are our most valuable treasures and they bestow us with the ability to enjoy human experiences, inspire others and change the world. We should always strive to engrave beautiful memories of ourselves and our legacy on the tree of life. Finally, you can never know what it feels like to be another person, so we should tolerate other people's afflictions to make them feel better. Don't treat such people poorly--instead, give them new pleasurable memories.

workout: none
☐ rest

cardio: none
☐ rest

nutrition:
☐ drink at least eight 8-ounce cups of water
☐ take a multivitamin
☐ eat only lean meats, fish, seafood, nuts, fruits and vegetables
☐ drink 1 serving of a protein shake before breakfast and dinner
☐ enjoy sugars, juice, sweets and soda in moderation
☐ avoid all artificially colored and processed foods

day ninety - three:
reinforcement

> The goal of life is living in agreement with nature.
> <u>Zeno</u>

Humans love fashion, and this is quite evident by the large number of magazines dedicated to designer clothes. Every season, many of us browse and study fashion magazines like someone searching for the world's next greatest invention. As a result we tend to be very knowledgeable of what's 'in" and what's 'out" of style. Aside from 'fashionability," it appears few people truly appreciate the value and importance of clothes. Have you ever noticed how most clothes are made from a bunch of flimsy threads? It's amazing how all those threads can entwine together to make a sturdy and durable piece of clothing. From experience, we know that a single cotton thread will break with the slightest force, so how come, say, jeans, which are made entirely from cotton, are so durable? To put it simply, all the threads add their individual strengths together. Similarly, many little ideas can combine to make great works for society. Think of all the books, scientific experiments, buildings and machines that came about after people shared and pursued their ideas. Every one of us has unique ideas that are capable of influencing and changing the world for the better. It is quite unfortunate, though, that many of these ideas (like a single cotton thread) are lost or broken because we never share them with other people or try to cultivate them. It is important to learn as much as you can about other people's ideas and share your own ideas with others. You never know, your ideas could be great by themselves or they could help someone else make a great discovery that benefits all of humanity. Always remember that a great mind along with its ideas is a terrible thing to waste.

---

workout: chest

☐ incline bench press   [10 reps x 5 times]

weights (lbs):					

☐ decline bench press   [10 reps x 5 times]

weights (lbs):					

☐ flat bench press   [10 reps x 5 times]

weights (lbs):					

☐ pec deck   [10 reps x 5 times]

weights (lbs):					

☐ hammer press   [10 reps x 5 times]

weights (lbs):					

☐ dips   [20 reps x 5 times]

weights (lbs):					

cardio: treadmill

☐ paced walk/jog   [30 minutes]

calories:	

nutrition:

☐ drink at least eight 8-ounce cups of water
☐ take a multivitamin
☐ eat only lean meats, fish, seafood, nuts, fruits and vegetables
☐ drink 1 serving of a protein shake before breakfast and dinner
☐ avoid starches, grains, sugars, juice, sweets and soda
☐ avoid all artificially colored and processed foods

day ninety - four:
gone astray

You always pass failure on the way to success.
Mickey Rooney

Have you ever been lost when driving someplace? It can be quite a harrowing experience, especially when the driving conditions are not optimal or when you are late for an important appointment. Once I drove to visit a friend and I became completely lost after it started pouring down rain and I took a few wrong turns. Frustrated yet resolute, I kept on driving in hopes that I would find the right road but I never came across it. Panic soon set in once I realized that I didn't have my phone to call for help. The more I drove through the city, the more unfamiliar the entire area appeared. Luckily, through the downpour, I found another gas station and asked the sales clerk for assistance. To my relief I discovered that I was only about a mile from my friend's house. Similar to driving, the feeling of being lost in life can be frustrating and overwhelming to the point that many of us feel like we are trapped in a maze with little to no guidance. The truth is that fear and panic can be great thieves of our joy and sanity. Like expert muggers, these emotional states are constantly on the prowl to exploit our weaknesses to bring us down to our knees. However, remaining calm during these trying times can save unneeded stress and grant us the mental clarity needed to tackle the obstacles in our way. Even wild animals have methods to navigate through dense woods, so we should also use our internal sense of direction (besides online maps!) to ensure that we're able to avoid getting lost. This may require goal-setting and studying 'maps" of the areas in life that you will like to explore so that you understand the 'big picture." Everyone has this internal sense of direction--we just have to develop it. It is important that you keep your cool, and if you do so you'll find yourself where you want to be.

tasks:

workout: back/traps

☐ deadlift   [10 reps x 5 times]

weights (lbs):					

☐ pulldowns   [10 reps x 5 times]

weights (lbs):					

☐ bent over row   [10 reps x 5 times]

weights (lbs):					

☐ cable row   [10 reps x 5 times]

weights (lbs):					

☐ pull ups   [10 reps x 5 times]

weights (lbs):					

☐ shrugs   [10 reps x 5 times]

weights (lbs):					

cardio: stairmaster

☐ paced walk   [30 minutes]

calories:	

nutrition:

☐ drink at least eight 8-ounce cups of water
☐ take a multivitamin
☐ eat only lean meats, fish, seafood, nuts, fruits and vegetables
☐ drink 1 serving of a protein shake before breakfast and dinner
☐ avoid starches, grains, sugars, juice, sweets and soda
☐ avoid all artificially colored and processed foods

Sheg Aranmolate, MD

day ninety - five:
flexible

> Adapt or perish, now as ever, is nature's inexorable
> imperative.
> H. G. Wells

We live in an ever-changing world of technologies, fashions and politics, and this requires us to constantly adapt. In a matter of a few years the way we communicate with others and access information has changed drastically with the explosion of the internet and other wireless communication technologies. Once, I saw a movie about a young man who had been sleeping for countless years in a cryogenic chamber, only to be awoken by a couple of curious boys. The movie had a romantic storyline that suggested that certain human emotions like affection, compassion, kindness and love are timeless. But the man had to adjust to an entirely different society filled with such changes as new modes of transportation and communication, new infrastructures, and new medicines, just to name a few. Can you imagine such a drastic change? Change in life and our society is inevitable as the young members grow to fill the positions of the old. As such, change can often be a nice and desirable experience. On the other hand, many of us sometimes get frustrated and even depressed following drastic changes in our lives. For instance, a young professional recently got promoted to a position that he had always wanted only to find out it was a bad fit for his personality and future ambitions. With new long hours and stressful demands from his boss, the job made him physically exhausted and emotionally drained to the point of depression, and at one point he was on the verge of suicide. The man's story teaches us to be careful about the changes we pursue because we may later regret such changes. Nevertheless, we all need to be flexible enough to accommodate change but resilient enough to withstand the impacts of the change. Always view change--no matter how drastic--as a golden opportunity to learn more about your inner strengths and weaknesses.

tasks:

workout: legs

☐ squats   [10 reps x 5 times]

weights (lbs):				

☐ squat to bench   [10 reps x 5 times]

weights (lbs):				

☐ quad extensions   [15 reps x 5 times]

weights (lbs):				

☐ leg curls   [15 reps x 5 times]

weights (lbs):				

☐ leg press calf raises   [20 reps x 5 times]

weights (lbs):				

☐ seated calf raises   [20 reps x 5 times]

weights (lbs):				

cardio: elliptical

☐ paced walk   [30 minutes]

calories:	

nutrition:

☐ drink at least eight 8-ounce cups of water
☐ take a multivitamin
☐ eat only lean meats, fish, seafood, nuts, fruits and vegetables
☐ drink 1 serving of a protein shake before breakfast and dinner
☐ avoid starches, grains, sugars, juice, sweets and soda
☐ avoid all artificially colored and processed foods

Sheg Aranmolate, MD

day ninety - six:
impenetrable thoughts

Any fool can criticize, condemn, and complain - and most fools do.
Dale Carnegie

Once I saw a television show about a street-savvy magician who awed pedestrians with different tricks. I was immediately intrigued because, as a kid, I was fond of Harry Houdini, a great magician, and I thought magic was real. Of course as I got older and wiser I came to the bitter realization that magical acts were simply illusions resulting from our flawed sensory system (our perception). Nevertheless, I watched the show to see if I could figure out the 'prestige" behind his acts and was impressed by their novelty, especially when he performed the seemingly impossible task of reading other people's thoughts. This trick was amazing because the human mind is like an impenetrable fortress that is filled with a diverse array of thoughts and ideas. We all share some commonality in our flawed perceptions of reality that, under the right conditions and state of mind, we can be deceived into believing things regardless of their veracity. Have you ever taken a moment to think about the way you think and the factors that influence your thought process? This might seem like a circular question, but the irrefutable truth is that the way we think determines the way we view the world. The ability to think and our possession of free will is one of our greatest assets as humans. It is much easier said than done but don't let other people trick you into believing anything. Suppose you're in a debate or argument with a stranger or even an associate, you shouldn't let yourself be dragged into fallacious reasoning, like when people try to convince you that something is true because a majority of people believe it to be true. In particular, be careful to not get caught up in all the talking points of great illusionists and distorters of the truth.

workout: deltoids

☐ military press behind the neck   [10 reps x 5 times]

weights (lbs):					

☐ military press   [10 reps x 5 times]

weights (lbs):					

☐ dumbbell shoulder press   [10 reps x 5 times]

weights (lbs):					

☐ machine shoulder press   [10 reps x 5 times]

weights (lbs):					

☐ reverse pec deck   [10 reps x 5 times]

weights (lbs):					

☐ dumbbell front raises   [20 reps x 5 times]

weights (lbs):					

cardio: treadmill

☐ paced walk/jog   [30 minutes]

calories:	

nutrition:

☐ drink at least eight 8-ounce cups of water
☐ take a multivitamin
☐ eat only lean meats, fish, seafood, nuts, fruits and vegetables
☐ drink 1 serving of a protein shake before breakfast and dinner
☐ avoid starches, grains, sugars, juice, sweets and soda
☐ avoid all artificially colored and processed foods

day ninety - seven:
artistic interpretation

> Opinions founded on prejudice are always sustained with the greatest of violence.
> Francis Jeffrey

The Mona Lisa is one of the most famous paintings by the great artist Leonardo da Vinci. It depicts a young lady gazing directly at the viewers with a countenance that lacks expression. Despite being a rather boring-looking painting, it has become the subject of much analysis and parody. There are numerous interpretations of the painting and many believe it has several religious, sexual and aesthetic overtones. This painting is particularly intriguing to me, not necessarily for its great artistic and aesthetic values, but because it reveals a lot about the way we judge and interpret our lives and the lives of others. Every one of us has a unique view of life that results from our biology and environment. Just as people have different interpretations of the Mona Lisa, we always have different accounts of the same incident, such as a party, a political debate or basketball game. Because of our subjective and dogmatic nature, many of us can be rather quick to criticize other people's interpretations and impose our subjective views and opinions on others. It is sad that many of us fail to realize that our opinions are sometimes incorrect and, similar to a toddler who clings onto his or her parents, many of us cling to our false opinions. However, this doesn't mean that we should ever abandon our values, principles, and opinions, but rather be willing to acknowledge the potential validity of other people's opinions. This open-mindedness will allow us to better understand people and this will in turn allow others to be more receptive to our unique views of the world.

workout: arms/forearms

☐ pushdowns   [10 reps x 5 times]

weights (lbs):					

☐ wide grip curls   [10 reps x 5 times]

weights (lbs):					

☐ single arm cable kickbacks   [10 reps x 5 times]

weights (lbs):					

☐ seated triceps press   [10 reps x 5 times]

weights (lbs):					

☐ hammer curls   [10 reps x 5 times]

weights (lbs):					

☐ concentration curls   [20 reps x 5 times]

weights (lbs):					

cardio: stairmaster

☐ paced walk   [30 minutes]

calories:	

nutrition:

☐ drink at least eight 8-ounce cups of water
☐ take a multivitamin
☐ eat only lean meats, fish, seafood, nuts, fruits and vegetables
☐ drink 1 serving of a protein shake before breakfast and dinner
☐ avoid starches, grains, sugars, juice, sweets and soda
☐ avoid all artificially colored and processed foods

day ninety - eight:
knowledgeable criticism

> If you are not criticized, you may not be doing much.
> Donald H. Rumsfeld

I am very particular about the movies I see in the theater because time is scarce and I only want to see great movies. Whenever there is a highly anticipated movie coming to the theater, I read the reviews of the movie from film critics. Movie reviews have rarely convinced me to watch a movie but instead have given me a clear sense of the plot. Nevertheless, over the years I have realized that, despite the subjective nature of movie criticisms, there is usually some level of truth to the critiques. Criticism is important for our growth and the growth of our society. For example, in the scientific world some of the world's greatest scientific breakthroughs and inventions have resulted from corrections made to previously criticized works. An example of this is in the development of the Polio vaccine, which has saved millions of children from the debilitating and deadly disease. Let's be honest with ourselves: many of us don't like to be criticized but we often love to criticize others. It is absurd that many of us are quick to find flaws or faults in others while being blind to our own flaws. We 'blind critics" may help others by pointing out their faults but we never improve ourselves in that manner. Criticized people usually repair their faults while many of us criticizers are left to wallow in ignorance of our many faults. Remember that the Oscar Awards and movie critics help consumers determine the quality of a movie. If there was a similar awards show or group of critiques for your attitudes and behavior, how well will you be rated? Please don't be one of those 'blind critics"-- it's ok to give constructive criticism of others, just accept correct criticism of yourself.

workout: abs/core

☐ weighted sit ups   [20 reps x 5 times]

weights (lbs):					

☐ weighted cable crunch   [10 reps x 5 times]

weights (lbs):					

☐ leg raises   [20 reps x 5 times]

weights (lbs):					

☐ air bike   [60 reps x 5 times]

weights (lbs):					

☐ side bends   [40 reps x 5 times]

weights (lbs):					

☐ hanging leg raises   [20 reps x 5 times]

weights (lbs):					

cardio: elliptical

☐ paced walk   [30 minutes]

calories:	

nutrition:

☐ drink at least eight 8-ounce cups of water
☐ take a multivitamin
☐ eat only lean meats, fish, seafood, nuts, fruits and vegetables
☐ drink 1 serving of a protein shake before breakfast and dinner
☐ avoid starches, grains, sugars, juice, sweets and soda
☐ avoid all artificially colored and processed foods

day ninety - nine:
the stock exchange

Take calculated risks. That is quite different from being rash.
George S. Patton

My parents used to be members of a number of medical, societal and charitable associations, and every year we would host a few meetings in our house. These gatherings were memorable because my beautiful mother would always cook an array of delicious foods for our guests and I would circle the dining room table like a vulture, impatiently waiting for the meetings to be over so that I could feast. As soon as the guests began to eat, they would often digress from their conversations about medicine and community service to talk about economics, retirement plans and the stock market. During these conversations, I learned much about the international stock market and when I got older I even began to follow it on my own. I have come to learn that the course of our lives can be similar to the stock market. For example, just as investors should learn about a company before investing in its stocks, we should best understand our strengths and weaknesses before we pursue our goals and tackle our aspirations in life. Also, just as investors are careful not to put too much money into a single stock position, we should be very cautious in placing all our hope in one goal. In addition, similar to investors managing diverse portfolios with both long and short-term investments, we also need to have backup plans along with long and short-term goals in our lives. This helps us maximize our successes in our endeavors and minimize our failures. We must realize that there's always a risk of failure. Nevertheless, taking calculated risks in life can be the difference between success and failure. As you navigate through life, it is important to be as knowledgeable as possible about any risks that you take in pursuit of success.

workout: none
□ rest

cardio: none
□ rest

nutrition:
□ drink at least eight 8-ounce cups of water
□ take a multivitamin
□ eat only lean meats, fish, seafood, nuts, fruits and vegetables
□ drink 1 serving of a protein shake before breakfast and dinner
□ enjoy sugars, juice, sweets and soda in moderation
□ avoid all artificially colored and processed foods

Sheg Aranmolate, MD

day one - hundred:
different kind of genius

> The secret to creativity is knowing how to hide your sources.
> Albert Einstein

The name 'Einstein"--that of one of the world's greatest physicists--has become synonymous with the word genius. He was a genius in the physical sciences; his scientific works answered some of the most challenging questions in physics and chemistry, such as the relationship between energy and the speed of light. Einstein never limited himself to the sciences and also made profound contributions to the liberal arts and world politics (e.g. denouncing the Nazi movement in Germany and participating in several civil rights movements). As a child, Einstein had a speech impediment and he also failed his first entrance exam into college. However, like most successful people he didn't give up and successfully reapplied. We live in a world where, for the most part, being different is condemned and conformity is praised. There are many of us who are afraid of our unique characteristics, such as our unique ideas and intellectual abilities, and try very hard to blend into the crowd. Have you ever heard the story of the ugly duckling? This 'duckling" was ostracized by other ducks because it looked strange-- later in life the ugly duckling transformed into a majestic swan. Just like the duckling, there are times when it is impossible for us to blend into the crowd and, during those times, it's important for us to let our differences shine. If great thinkers like Einstein had decided to ignore their unique ideas, then we might not be enjoying many of our luxuries and technologies. Please don't be scared to share your unique characteristics--they may make a lasting contribution to humanity. At the very least, sharing your uniqueness will bring you happiness and may help people around you.

tasks:

workout: none
- ☐ rest

cardio: none
- ☐ rest

nutrition:
- ☐ drink at least eight 8-ounce cups of water
- ☐ take a multivitamin
- ☐ eat only lean meats, fish, seafood, nuts, fruits and vegetables
- ☐ drink 1 serving of a protein shake before breakfast and dinner
- ☐ enjoy sugars, juice, sweets and soda in moderation
- ☐ avoid all artificially colored and processed foods

progress:
- ☐ take a full body photo on day 100
- ☐ record your weight and calculate your BMI (body mass index)

day one (1):	weight (lbs):		BMI:	
day one-hundred(100):	weight (lbs):		BMI:	
net difference:	weight (lbs):		BMI:	

- ☐ compare your full body photo on day 1 with day 100
- ☐ share your awesome transformation with friends and family

#congratulations ! ! !

Sheg Aranmolate, MD

The End!

'The end of one opportunity is the beginning of two new opportunities: to learn from the past and to create the future."

- Sheg Aranmolate -
☺

Thank you for reading and please help spread the word!

about the author:

Sheg Aranmolate considers himself an amateur polymath but definitely not a genius of any sort. He earned a bachelor's degree in Biochemistry and Molecular Biology with a minor in Psychology from the University of Maryland, where he pioneered a biweekly fitness column in the college newspaper, The Retriever Weekly. He also earned a master's degree in Applied Molecular Biology from the University of Maryland, and a doctorate degree in Medicine from the University of Tennessee. He completed an internship in General Surgery, and he is currently honing his business skills as he pursues a master's degree in Business Administration from the University of Texas. He holds a patent for potential anti-microbial compounds and his published indie novel, Bountiful Famine, was nominated for the IMPAC Dublin Literary Award. When not spending time with his wife and kids or musing about the world's greatest mysteries, he is hitting the gym or dreaming about eating sushi.

INSPIVIA

www.ingramcontent.com/pod-product-compliance
Lightning Source LLC
Chambersburg PA
CBHW071119280326
41935CB00010B/1059